Praise for Lou Paget's
Exquisitely Pleasurable
Techniques

THE MEN SAY . . .

"I already knew five languages, but tonight after your seminar I now consider myself a cunnilinguist."

Executive, 54, Pasadena

"I had no idea this subject area could be treated with such grace and elegance while still delivering an informed and powerful message. You have a most unique seminar."

German documentary director, 58, Paris

"I saw the results of your presentation at my bachelor dinner. The next night, on the dance floor after our wedding, my friends and their wives were dancing closer, kissing and hugging more *and* the wives couldn't stop thanking me. Thank you!"

Publisher, 42, Indianapolis

"*Finally!* The information we guys have always wanted and women haven't told us. Anytime I can learn more about my woman and how to please her, sign me up, and it just hasn't been available like this before and it's good to get it from their gender perspective."

Radio talk show host, 44, New Jersey

"I learned more in three hours at your seminar than I did in my two previous marriages."

Systems engineer, 47, Chicago

"It is surprising to me that men do not have as much arrogance about learning about money as they do about learning about sex. A man can always talk about ways to make more $ yet underneath the one thing he really wants to know how to do best is 'make it' with his partner."

Accountant, 51, Denver

"I had no idea how little idea I had—I thank you and my fiancée thanks you."

Novelist, 42, Santa Monica

"Thank you, thank you, thank you! Do you know what a gold mine you are? Every man, teenager, college student, whatever, should have access to your course."

Attorney, 32, New York

"After my brother and I had attended your class we could talk more freely and not just in the way guys usually do. I think your message about respecting our sexuality was the biggest one for me."

College student, 25, St. Louis

"It was the simplest of things, it was the ways you showed me how to stroke and touch my wife. I only wish I had known this forty years ago."

Recently married executive, 64, Beverly Hills

"I read the Kama Sutra when I was fourteen or fifteen and it made about as much sense as Bobby Fischer's book on chess moves—and

I could just see an old guy with a heart condition trying this stuff having a heart attack in the garage on the third day. Thank God we finally have you as a source of information."

Photographer, 47, Oakland

THEIR PARTNERS SAY

"Lou, this is G's wife, he did your seminar last week. And what can I say, I am yet another *satisfied* customer."

Author, 47, Manhattan

"We had adopted our first child and then we each did your seminar. Three months later I got pregnant and I want you to know my husband and I hold you completely responsible for our beautiful baby girl."

Singer/actress, 36, Encino

"You put the spark back into a forty-year marriage—something we had hoped for and can't believe has actually happened."

Retail executive, 63, Las Vegas

"I am amazed at how comfortable we are about talking about sexual things now. After the class my husband of fifteen years said, 'You know what, I really want to talk and we did!' We found out things we both wanted to do and try and had never had the courage to ask—are we having fun."

Producer, 41, Phoenix

"At first I thought he can't get better or know more; he was already a fabulous lover. But there was something about what he heard from you that gave him the permission or I don't know what that moved our sex life from good to great to amazing. We now connect sexually even better in our bodies and at a much deeper level in our hearts."

Full-time housewife, 52, Minneapolis

"It is almost embarrassing how obvious the results of my husband's seminar are on me. If one more friend asks me why I look so good— I'll just laugh and say my husband took a class."

Marketing executive, 28, San Francisco

How to Give Her Absolute Pleasure

Also by Lou Paget

HOW TO BE A GREAT LOVER

HOW TO GIVE HER

ABSOLUTE

· PLEASURE

TOTALLY EXPLICIT TECHNIQUES
EVERY WOMAN WANTS
HER MAN TO KNOW

Lou Paget

Broadway Books / NEW YORK

BROADWAY

Broadway Books titles may be purchased for business or promotional
use or for special sales. For information, please write to:
Special Markets Department, Random House, Inc.,
1540 Broadway, New York, NY 10036.

BROADWAY BOOKS and its logo, a letter B bisected on the diagonal,
are trademarks of Broadway Books, a division
of Random House, Inc.

Visit our Web site at www.broadwaybooks.com

Library of Congress Cataloging-in-Publication Data
Paget, Lou.
How to give her absolute pleasure: totally explicit techniques
every woman wants her man to know / Lou Paget—1st. ed.
p. cm.
1. Sex instruction for men. 2. Women—Sexual behavior.
3. Men—Sexual behavior. 4. Sexual excitement. I. Title.
HQ36.P34 2000
613.9'6—dc21   99-047769

FIRST EDITION

DESIGNED BY JENNIFER ANN DADDIO

ISBN 0-7679-0452-4

00   01   02   03   04   10   9   8   7   6

*To my father, Kenneth Kane Paget, the first man
I ever loved with all my heart.*

&

*To all of the gentlemen in the seminars, who had the
courage to say what you wanted. You planted the seed.
To all of the gentlemen and ladies who shared their ideas.
You gave the book its soul and direction.
To all of the gentlemen who asked for this book.
You are the reason it came into being.*

Acknowledgments

_____ • _____

One of the things you learn when you are involved in any project is that no one does it alone, and one of the sweeter things is to let those who have been there for you know how much you appreciate them.

THE SUPPORT TEAM
The ladies in my family who once again were always there: Dede, Katerena, Sherry, Lisa, Michelle, and Carolynn.

Tara Raucci, my ever-capable assistant, who hit the ground running.

Jessica Kalkin, Bernard Spigner (my "NP"), Matthew Davidge, Maura McAniff, Kendra King, Raymond Davi, T. J. Rozsa, Priscilla Wallace, Sandra Beck, Jay Rosen, Alan Cochran, Michael Levin, Nance Mitchell, Peter Redgrove, Morley Winnick, Gail Harrington, Elizabeth Hall, Eileen Michaels, Robert McGarvey, Mark Helm, Lilianna and Ali Moradi.

THE REVIEW TEAM
Bernard Spigner, Matthew Davidge, Michael Levin, Marty Waldman, Rafi Tahmazian, Ron Ireland, Wayne Williams, David James, T. J. Rozsa, Jay Rosen, Craig Dellio.

THE CREATIVE TEAM

Billie Fitzpatrick, who again took my voice and masterfully turned it into words. A West Coast to East Coast production, you can only imagine our e-mails.

Debra Goldstein, the agent every author dreams of . . . pats to Bodhi.

Lauren Marino, an editor with the guts to truly edit, to do so stylishly, and, into book two (with me and Billie), she still has one of the best laughs.

Ann Campbell, associate editor; Cate Tynan, editorial assistant; Bill Betts, copy editor; "J," the illustrator; Andrea Thomas, the graphic artist for the cover.

All at Broadway Books and the Creative Culture.

THE RESEARCH AND DEVELOPMENT TEAM

Penelope Hitchcock, D.V.M., Stephen Sacks, M.D., Beverly Whipple, Ph.D., Laura Berman, Ph.D., Linda Banner, M.S., Jacqueline Snow, M.N., C.N.P., Bernie Zilbergeld, Ph.D., Bryce Britton, M.S., Dennis Paradise, Eric Daar, M.D., Michael Loring Probst.

Contents

———— • ————

———— • ————

ONE

The Yin and the Yang
of the KamaLoutra

You Asked for It

I can still remember when I first realized how frustrated men were about sex. The turning point was one particular night about four years ago. It was a Saturday in late May, and I had just arrived at a friend's house for a dinner party. I had been tied up in traffic on the freeway and was the last guest to arrive. I was already tired and had lost my enthusiasm for the party, making an effort to be polite, charming, and upbeat. I sat down next to a gentleman who looked to be in his early forties and introduced myself. We got to talking and he told me that he was a television producer. He then asked what I did. For a moment, I felt myself begin to blush, and then I went for it. I should not have felt embarrassed or hesitant to say what I do after having done it for three years at that point, but I had found myself already feeling a bit shy. I then said to him, as demurely as possible, "Well, I give sex seminars to women." Without skipping a beat, he looked straight at me and asked, "Well, do you give them to men, too? We need them!"

In an instant it dawned on me that men, like women, are not only curious about sex, but feel confined or restricted by what they know and do not know. The more I began to listen and talk to men, the more I realized that most men seem to think and feel that they are expected to *already* know everything there is to know about sex, as if the information is tied to their Y chromosome, which neatly and completely surfaces with the first hair on their chin. The more I thought about it, I realized that men are actually acculturated to know *all* about sex—what works well, feels the best—both for themselves and for the women they're with. Whereas it's all right for women not to know, many men feel enormous pressure to possess an encyclopedic knowledge of all things sexual. This is not only an enormous falsehood but also an unfair burden for men.

The solution to this problem is simple. First, men need to be granted the permission to ask questions about what they don't know or are not comfortable with regarding sex. Second, and perhaps more important, men need to realize that all women are different and therefore require different treatment. There is no possible way to know what works best for a woman without asking her. Finally, men need to realize that the onus of sex does not fall solely on men. Both men and women should be responsible for learning and then knowing about how to please one another. If these factors are in place, any man can become an expert lover.

I've been curious about sex since I was a teenager, but it took me almost twenty years to gain enough confidence and knowledge to feel comfortable speaking about how to be a great lover. As a woman, my dilemma was that there was no apparent way to be both a nice girl and one that knew a lot about sex. When I realized I was curious about sex, I also realized that there was no safe, dependable source of information I could access. My girlfriends knew only limited amounts about sexuality. And sleeping around wasn't a reasonable or respectable option. So after I surveyed the porn magazines, the movies, and various books on the subject, including the *Kama Sutra*, *The Joy of Sex*, and *The Sensuous Woman*, I came up fairly empty-handed. There was no one source that gave me what I was looking for: accurate, complete information about sex. Consequently, I began talking, asking questions, and then sharing information about sexual experiences with my women friends. It was from and through them that I began to learn what works, what turns men on, and what doesn't. After all, who is better to say what works than someone who knows what works for them?

Soon I found myself an amateur sexpert simply because I felt it was important and necessary that accurate, reliable information about sex be available to all women—whatever their age, background, or experience. I had gathered the stories and details of the women who had shared with me and began assembling and presenting the information to focus groups, which then gave me feedback. To make a long story very short, that's how the sex seminars for women were born.

Not surprisingly, as soon as these women returned to their husbands, boyfriends, or partners, I began receiving calls, suggestions, and then pleas from men to "please, please, if you're doing this for women, you have to do it for us, too." So in the same way that I created the seminars to teach women about their bodies, men's bodies, and what the two can do together to experience sex in the most passionate ways possible, I began my quest to do the same for men. Over the course of the last six years, I have interviewed and shared information with literally thousands of men and women. That's how both the men's seminars and this book were born.

The men's seminar is a group of six to ten men, introduced only by first name, not by surname or by what they do. At a big round table I distribute to each man an "instructional product," which is a life-size woman's genitalia made of a soft, fleshlike material molded from a porn star. Without too much fanfare, I show the attendees what works for women and what doesn't—manually, orally, during penetration, how women most often reach orgasm, and what toys to use that will drive women wild in bed. This information is based on the data I've gathered from my field researchers.

The men who attend my seminars have been all types—professionals, artists, athletes, doctors, mechanics, architects, builders, actors, producers, television executives. They have come in all sizes and shapes, education levels, and personalities. And they have all come wanting to know more about sex—specifically, how better to please the women in their lives. As one political consultant said, "Making love makes me feel manly, in the most basic sense of the word. There is nothing that makes sex with my partner better than knowing I can take care of her. So if there is information out there for me to experience that more and differently, then I want it." Another seminar attendee, this one an investment banker from New York, said he wanted this book for another reason. Referring to his wife, he put it this way: "We've been together ten years and I want to know how to make it more fun, more interesting." Another male seminar attendee, a photographer from Palo Alto, California, said, "Please, just tell me what works."

I hear not only yearning in these voices but a demand for the tried-and-true. A real estate developer from Philadelphia said in frustration, "I wouldn't ask her to do anything she doesn't want to do, but I'd love to know anything that is going to make our sex life keep growing. It is good, really good, but I want to make it better."

This book was created for you, gentlemen, because you deserve it. Besides, how could I resist the slow, rising din of men (the boyfriends, the husbands, the partners) yearning for a book about how to give absolute pleasure to the women in their lives? So here it is: You asked for it, you got it.

Becoming an Expert Lover

My work these past seven years giving the sexuality seminars to both men and women has taught me a great deal about male and female sexuality as well as their psychology. The information in this book, then, comes from my listening and observing and hearing the feed-back that thousands of men and women share with me about what works, what doesn't, and what they're missing. Don't you want to know what women honestly want, like, and don't like? I want to be your special confidante, a translator and provider of women's hidden desires and wishes. Inside these two covers, I have assembled—for her benefit as well as yours—the most scintillating, most practical, and most reliable information out there. If you believe that one's sexual prowess is gained by being with skilled, sensitive, and informative lovers, think of this book as that one lover who will share all she knows—and she knows a lot!

Another way to think of me is as your coach. In sports it's perfectly understandable and acceptable to have a coach, as it is in business to have a mentor. While I don't pretend to be a doctor of sex, I do think that my so-called time in the field, gathering information from thousands of men and women, has enabled me to present you with what works best in the sex department for both women and men. I presume that you are tired of the same old, stale information that purports to give you the real goods but falls short. Rather, I think you ultimately want to know what works, what's going to warm her up, get her excited, and eventually have her scream your name in ecstasy. I will describe the tips to perfect your "game" and point out snafus that may hinder your giving her *absolute pleasure*. I'm going to tell it like it is, from the point of view of women, and I'm not going to spare you any details. I feel confident that, as your coach, I will not lead you astray, but rather will lead you down the path to mutual bliss.

This book is the first step in making you an expert lover. How does one become an expert? In order to transform yourself from a competent lover to one who can bring his lover to unparalleled heights of pleasure, you must not only learn the tried-and-true techniques of a master seducer but also incorporate the insight that makes you open, willing, and ready to climb such heights.

How to Give Her Absolute Pleasure is about how to please women, pamper them, and thrill them. So I'm making another assumption here: that you, the readers, not only want to be on the top of your sexual game but also care deeply and passionately about women. And although the women in your lives will be the direct beneficiaries of the treasure trove of information between these seductive covers, doesn't it make sense that by pleasing your partner, you will receive that pleasure back in spades? Sex, like other endeavors, whether they are career-oriented, spiritual, physical, or emotional, is about synergy. Specifically, if you please your partner, her satisfaction builds and bounces back to you, increasing your pleasure. As one physician from Seattle said, "There is nothing that is better than knowing I have taken care of her, that I made her feel great. That for me is what making love is all about." Another man said, "Like most guys, I do not want people knowing what I do with my wife at those most intimate moments. And even though women may talk about sex, we men don't or can't. But my male pride went into orbit when my wife told me that I had become the guy her friends wanted cloned and who they talk about in *their* locker room!"

SECRET FROM LOU'S ARCHIVES
The use of lipstick apparently originates from wanting to have the oral labia resemble the blood-flushed look of the aroused genital labia. In the animal kingdom this indicates to the male that the female is sexually ready.

In preparing and doing the seminars, I discovered that reliable or accurate sources of information about sex are very limited. The typical sources men use to learn about sex are slanted and incomplete. Male pornography—both magazines and films—is problematic for three main reasons. First, the majority of porn magazines and movies are created with the visual stimulation/fantasy factor as the driving force and are therefore often unrealistic. Second, because they "program" men to expect the unrealistic in sex, men are disappointed when women or their bodies can't or don't deliver. Third, because these movies and magazines are targeted to men, they ignore half the population (i.e., women), which means that what pleases women is not adequately or faithfully represented.

Although I have nothing against visual material that stimulates men, I think it's important to know that while some of these fantasies may work in your mind to get you excited, they may not work in real life. By all means, use these movies, written scenarios, or other forms of pornography to pleasure you and even your partner. I know one seminar attendee and his partner who loved to read each other some of the erotica stories in *Playboy*. He said, "Sometimes it just helps to get us in the mood." But when these scenarios are actually brought into the bedroom and acted out, many men and women are often surprised, frustrated, and ultimately disappointed when they don't work.

Remember, these are actors—professionals—who are working on choreographed sets with props, editing, voice-overs, and special lighting, which all combine to create an unreal environment. If a fantasy story of one man making love with two women is a turn-on for you (and perhaps your partner as well), things may get a bit more complicated when such a scenario is 'tested' in real life. Real feelings are at stake, and no matter how open one or both of you may be in terms of your fantasies, you may end up getting hurt, the intimacy and trust between you and your partner forever severed. I asked a television talk show host what he felt was the basis for porn, and he said, "Minimal plot ideas with the aim to get the clothes off as soon as possible and get into the action, geared at men aged seventeen to thirty-seven."

Another downfall of relying too heavily on porn and the fantasies they promote is that they tend to program men to expect a certain kind of turn-on. Again, this expectation is rarely met in the real world. If your lover is unable to play out the fantasies as they are depicted or described in the movies or magazines, porn can actually distract and/or come between you and her. A good example of this is the frequency with which "deep throating," swallowing, or anal play appears in pornography. Again, while the images may stimulate or titillate you, many women cannot deep-throat and prefer not to swallow or be penetrated anally. Of course, there are women who love anal sex and the sensation of your semen down their throats. But from what thousands of women have shared with me, many women would rather not engage in these activities. Specifically, the gag reflex makes it nearly impossible to deep-throat. Again, the women in the films who are performing such feats are professionals, who do such moves day in, day out for the camera, not for a man they love or care about. Based on my seminars and research, I would say only 20 to 25 percent of women swallow, and although many women try anal sex at least once, most say it's too painful to be enjoyable.

In addition, I know of several people (a couple of men and one woman) who wrote for Larry Flynt publications' "personal experience" columns. They admitted that the published scenarios are completely made up. When I asked one gentleman, he said, "Lou, it was great fun writing those columns. I had a great time!" Yet in response to my question about how much of the information was truthful, he said, "Not a word." The same writer also wrote a first-person column on how to seduce and have sex with women in different countries. He went into great detail on the clubs, bars, and lounges where one could get the best action across Europe. A minor overlooked fact, however, was that this gentleman had never been out of the United States in his life. You got it: He made it all up.

Another source of misinformation about sex comes from that eponymous group called the "guys." In the seminars, men will often share the "helpful" information of friends. What they soon realize is that their friends don't know any more than they do; they just act like they do. As a rule, and many of you have probably already figured this out by now, the biggest talkers are usually the least informed. These are the locker-room braggarts who exaggerate in quantity and exploit the quality. As one man I know recalls, "This dude had eight guys listening to him brag about doing this married babe six times in one afternoon. Even though we knew he was full of sh——, we all were standing around like maybe some of that would fall off on us." Sound familiar?

Another gentleman I know stopped his twenty-three-year-old nephew's manly adventure story during the family picnic. When the nephew said, "Yeah, I did her eight times last night," the uncle said, "Okay, drop trou. Let's see it—that will be the proof. You should be so sore today you can't pee." As you can imagine, the nephew did not drop trou, but he did quickly drop the subject.

SECRET FROM LOU'S ARCHIVES
Women want variety but not necessarily performance; they aren't machines with off/on buttons and they don't come with manuals—although this book is, we hope, the next best thing.

Finally, pornography ignores half the population. The porn producers are there to make money—plain and simple. Until the bottom line is negatively affected by marketing only to men, these publishers and producers will keep churning out what customers seem to want. Why consider what women want if they don't have to? That said, there are a few producers who keep the female market in mind. One of these more female-friendly producers is Femme Productions, headed by Candida Royale. *The Wise Woman's Guide to Erotic Videos*, by Angela Cohen and Sarah Gardner Fox, is an excellent reference guide.

Sex as Performance

An indirect consequence of the problem with pornography is its dangerous reinforcement of sex as some kind of performance. Men look at the taut, muscular, never-aging bodies on-screen or in high-gloss print and automatically compare (and contrast) themselves. Although I know some of you can easily stand up to such scrutiny, I know even the most confident men may feel a bit put-off by the hard bodies displayed on-screen or in magazines. (The media do the same brainwashing on women when they use prepubescent women to model and when they airbrush and retouch advertisements.) No wonder you guys associate sex with pressure! The media are constantly reminding you to compare yourselves to the alpha males in magazines. I understand that most males have the basic trait of competitiveness, but for industry to manipulate this trait and use it to sell magazines or movies is just plain Machiavellian. Isn't this merely an exploitative business tactic of knowingly feeding the other side false information to gain competitive advantage? Best said, it is beyond unkind to force you to compare yourselves to false measurements and information.

Isn't a woman who really lets go and gets into sex a complete turn-on for you? Well, the same goes for women. Women don't want you to perform in bed. Nor do they necessarily care how many times you can "do it" in one night. Rather, they want you to enjoy being with them.

SECRET FROM LOU'S ARCHIVES

Always tell a woman what works, not what doesn't. Emphasize the positive and she'll listen.

If you are completely present, focused on her, and into what you're doing, a woman will not only feel cared for, she will also begin to unleash her sexual energy. As one seminar attendee told me, "The most satisfying sex happens in one long, slow lovemaking session."

The Communication Conundrum

We've all heard it over and over again: Men and women communicate differently. The king of communication between the sexes, John Gray, goes so far as saying that men access love through sex, while women access sex through love or feelings. If you ascribe to this theory, it's no wonder that men and women often find they're not speaking the same language. Haven't you ever felt that you and the woman in your life are speaking similar but not identical dialects, requiring a translator?

I won't bore you with an involved sociological study here, but suffice it to say that since boys and girls are socialized differently, based in general on their biology and then later reinforced by societal gender roles, they tend to communicate differently, in almost opposing ways. As a result, in order to communicate successfully—whether the subject is sex or dinner—I think it's important for men (and women) to acknowledge the differences between them. For instance, when a woman doesn't feel she's been heard, she will withdraw—both emotionally and physically. She may be reacting to you. As one woman said, "I fell in love with my husband when I discovered he absolutely listened. I couldn't believe it when days later he would consistently repeat what I had said, and understood where I was coming from—amazing."

Women respond best to the more self-confident and self-assured men, and those are men who listen. If a woman comes to you with a question, worry, concern, problem, or simple story from her life, she may not be asking for your advice. Ask her up front if she wants you to just listen or, if she does want advice, listen first and then give advice. Often she quite simply wants to be heard, and your listening means that you care. However, as a man, you may respond by wanting to "fix" her problem. Providing a solution isn't what she wants, and she may think you're being condescending. And if you constantly interrupt her while she is speaking, she will know you're not listening. Then she will withdraw, and where will that get either of you?

There are ways to communicate that you are listening to her: direct eye contact, touching her, and even a gentle nod of the head. If your eyes are darting all over the place, chances are you're not really paying attention, and chances are for sure that she knows you are distracted. And as I said above, when a woman doesn't feel heard, she will withdraw, both emotionally and physically, or find someone else who will listen. This is not a threat, just a fact. It is extremely important to women that they feel heard. One of their biggest complaints is that they aren't.

In the sexual arena, some gender differences in communicating have concrete effects or consequences. On the one hand, women want you to know what pleases them sexually; on the other hand, they are often reluctant to share this information with you in a direct way. Though women may talk among themselves about sex, many tend to shy away from talking directly to men about sex. This contrast points not only to a built-in communication challenge but also to these differences between men and women.

From my work in the seminars, I've narrowed down the four main reasons women hesitate to share what we want with our partners.

1. If we say what we want, we will be judged either as sleazy or as sexual traffic cops.
2. We don't know what to say or how to say it. A graphic designer from Miami said, "I'd love to tell him, I just don't know how. I know the sensation, but it's hard to describe exactly what he's doing to me."
3. We are concerned that men will feel criticized and hear our suggestions as a message that they aren't good lovers.
4. We are worried that men don't really listen. One woman said, "Even if I tell him what I like, he doesn't listen. He just keeps doing the same thing."

The reason some women won't tell you what they want or how to do it is related to one of those old stereotypes, which still has lingering power on female psyches. Most women, especially those who are single, often still want to be thought of as "nice girls," and don't want to risk being perceived as having slept around. They are afraid that men will hear any kind of "I like it this way" as an indication of what worked with "another guy." If they risk introducing this information, they fear that their partner may feel alienated or angry.

By being aware that women are hesitant to tell you their likes and dislikes, you can make the task of finding out what your partner wants simpler and easier (and far more pleasurable) for both of you if you tell her that you *want* to know. You need to encourage her to feel free to tell you, even show you at times, the way she wants to be touched, kissed, or licked, perhaps. By opening this front door of communication, you immediately establish a potent force for her relaxation.

Also, gentlemen, please be aware of how you deliver information. If you and your partner are comfortable with the term "pussy" and its various derivations, by all means use it. But know that if a woman is uncomfortable with the way you may describe *any* piece of her anatomy, chances are she will be turned off, not turned on. My suggestion here is to start with the most politically correct terms and go from there. You may want to ask her what she prefers to call her body parts, in conversation and in passion, and then adjust accordingly. Let her set the level of frankness. In other words, she may enjoy and get excited by using "dirty" words.

After being with the same lover for a long time, you can anticipate what she wants as well as surprise and explore with her, but if you're wondering how to please your lover consistently, then you need to communicate. There's just no way around it.

The importance of communication cannot be underestimated. Indeed, when you are conscious and aware of how you are interacting with her and how she is interacting with you, then all the other elements of sex will fall into place. As one male seminar attendee commented, "When you are with a woman, you have to be super, super aware. You have to forget about getting your rocks off and, instead, tune into her. The directions are right there for what she wants—you just have to pay total attention to what and how she reacts. She's like a schematic and you just need to adjust your hardwiring." With that in mind, I have put together a list of typical differences between men and women that you might want to keep in mind as you prepare yourself to become an expert lover. These, of course, are generalizations, and are not true for all men and women, but as a rule, they may be helpful.

- ➤ Women fall in love between their ears and men through their eyes.
- ➤ Men often enjoy a fast rush to sex. Women prefer a slow buildup.
- ➤ Men are goal-oriented, tending to head for the charge of orgasm. Women love the route getting there, meandering and taking their time.
- ➤ Most men absolutely love getting a wet, slippery tongue kiss in the ear, but most women abhor this. As one woman put it, "I feel my head is in a washing machine."
- ➤ Women respond to gentle, light touching. Men respond to deeper pressure.
- ➤ Women usually know when they are going to have sex, whereas men can be surprised. Women usually make up their minds based on how they've been treated. And often the thing that tips the tables isn't anything you are aware of. However, to put the odds more in your favor, we have written this book. The more you know, the better prepared you will be.
- ➤ Men tend to be visual creatures, coming alive at the mere sight of a bare breast. Women are more aural and tactile. They need to hear and to feel a man in order to get excited.

The Golden Parachute

Like any kind of project or endeavor, the more you put into sex, the more you and your lover will get out of it. Those men who say they have strong, wonderful, passionate love lives are those that approach sex with the same determination and gusto as they do their other goals, whether those goals are about their careers, artistic pursuits, humanitarian endeavors, or athletic interests. The consistent factor is focus. An oil executive from Arizona said, "When my sexual relationship and personal life are working well, I feel invincible in business. There is a direct correlation between being happy at home and being a success in my career." Again and again I've heard men say that when they are able to satisfy and fulfill their partner sexually, they feel better about themselves, more confident and energized in other areas of their lives.

In the same way that you plan ahead for your Saturday golf game, you need to plan for intercourse. In the beginning of a relationship, didn't you make more of an effort to seduce her? Well, don't forget this once you've been together for a while. No matter what your age or the status of your relationship, you still need to think ahead and make a commitment to your intimacy: Like your chip shot, your sexual relationship needs practice and concentration. I would bet that you have a long-term plan for your investments. How you take care of your money now affects its performance in the future. The same is true with your relationship: How you invest in your sexual relationship now pays off in the future. So you need to have a plan for your relationship as well. And believe me, you'll see very real returns.

If you've never put into words how sex connects you with her, let your partner know. Don't assume she knows exactly how you feel about the sex, intimacy, and connection. As one seminar attendee said, "I just assumed my wife knew how she turned me on. But after sex one time, she finally exploded and told me that she felt like all I wanted to do was f— her, and that I didn't love her. Nothing could be further from the truth, but I guess I thought she knew I loved her. Boy, was I wrong."

As you read through this book, I would like you to remember that I am sharing what I have learned and gleaned from the thousands of men and women I have encountered in my sexuality seminars. It goes without saying that all of these people attend the seminars in the spirit of mutual respect and wanting to learn how to be a great lover. And being a great lover is 20 percent technique and 80 percent openness, willingness, enthusiasm, and communication. That said, I want to thank you for being here. As I say to the men who walk through the door, sit down at an oval table among ten or so other men to hear about the techniques to best please ladies, it takes courage just to show up. But what you are about to receive may very well change your sex life forever.

Remember, there is no one window of opportunity for learning about sex. As we know, urban myths can carry the weight of the truth, yet like all myths, they shrink under direct scrutiny. The ultimate focus and goal of both the men's seminar and this book is to find and access your sexual soul. To give you the ideas, attitudes, and information that others say have worked for them so that as a lover, you can create a wondrous, playful, mutually enjoyable sexual relationship with the woman you love.

———— • ————

TWO

Safe Sensuality: Keeping You and Your Lady Protected

Knowledge Is Power

Safe sex doesn't have to mean boring sex. On the contrary, I like to think of it as a challenge to be creative. It's also a call for you to be considerate not only of your partner's comfort and protection but of your own as well. Bringing the subject of safety into your relationship can be a way of saying, "I care about you, I care about us." Furthermore, feeling protected, comfortable, and well taken care of is a crucial foundation for having great sex.

I realize this information is mainly needed by those people who are single and/or with new partners. However, before married people or those in long-term, committed relationships ignore this chapter, let me remind you that with the divorce rate being what it is, we should all be careful and forewarned—to some degree, even the most married among us experience some serial monogamy. For those of you who are parents, these facts are just as crucial. You may not want to scare your children, but you do want to do what parents do best and give your children information that prepares them for life, and sexually transmitted diseases (STDs) and sex are a part of life. You may want to consider two new statistics: first, that the average age of those newly infected by HIV has dropped from twenty-six to twenty; and second, that one in five people living with HIV were infected as teenagers.

What I have assembled in this chapter is the most up-to-date and accurate information regarding precautions and risk factors in having sex. It is crucial that you know what diseases are out there, what the figures are, and what you can and should do to prevent contraction. I understand that reminding you of the dangers may temporarily mute your sexual desire, but I trust you'll thank me later. Better your desire be extinguished for a few moments than have your sex life in the long term or even your life extinguished because of ignorance.

SECRET FROM LOU'S ARCHIVES
According to a recent study of Seattle teenagers, 80 percent of eighteen-year-old girls and 90 percent of eighteen-year-old boys were already sexually active. Sixty percent of those sexually active youths had had five or more partners. (Dr. Penelope Hitchcock, Chief of Sexually Transmitted Diseases Bureau of the National Institutes of Health)

In this day and age, safety is essential. It would be irresponsible of me to offer advice on sexual interaction without discussing safety first. To begin with, you may be surprised to know that as a man you are typically at less risk than your lady for contracting a sexually transmitted disease. Why is your lady at greater risk? It is partly a square-footage issue. Women have more mucosal tissue in the vaginal barrel than men do in the urethra of their penis. A second reason is that since women are typically the receptive partner during sex, and your body fluids are left *inside* her, she is more vulnerable to infection. The tissue most at risk during sexual encounters is the highly vascularized mucosal tissue of the vulva and vaginal barrel (for men this tissue is in the urethra) because it is easily abraded during sex. The corollary for women being more at risk is the need for men to take on greater responsibility to keep both of you safe. I know of a man who, upon entering a relationship, struggled with telling his new love about having herpes. Although she wasn't thrilled with his news, she very much appreciated his being honest and straightforward. She said it actually brought them closer. He was scrupulous about his hygiene and vigilant about any possible outbreaks. He also insisted on using condoms even when his lesions were inactive, and he avoided intercourse when they were. Meanwhile, he took suppressive antiviral therapy to reduce asymptomatic shedding. They've been together for six years and she has never developed herpes.

Now, before you think you don't have to worry about getting infected, think again. Ever gamble on low odds and won? From what I've observed in my seminars and other research, I've come to realize that many men assume that they are practicing safer sex when they (or their partners) use birth control. Safer sex is not merely about precautions against unwanted pregnancy. You must realize not only that it is, in part, your responsibility to use protection against pregnancy, but also that you are still at risk of becoming infected by an STD. Men as well as women can very often be asymptomatic of disease. In other words, you may not show any physical symptoms of being infected by a number of sexually transmitted diseases, but you can suffer long-term damage and can unknowingly pass on infection. This is especially true of chlamydia, human papilloma virus (HPV), and herpes (see below for more specific information on these and other diseases). So feeling well and not noticing a problem with your penis does not mean that you do not have a dangerous STD. Also be aware that the older you are, the greater the likelihood you are with a partner with a sexual history, and chances are people will "adjust" the details of their sexual history. So please be cautious and take the necessary preventive measures.

SECRET FROM LOU'S ARCHIVES

There is no absolutely "safe" period for sexual intercourse insofar as conception is concerned. Mother Nature is no fool in this regard. When a woman is highly sexually stimulated, she can ovulate out of cycle.

It wasn't too long ago that the term "safer sex" referred strictly to being kept safe from an unwanted pregnancy. And yet there is still misunderstanding in this area. As a forty-nine-year-old Episcopalian minister said, "Oh Lord, we used the rhythm method, and after our third unintended pregnancy, my wife and I thought we couldn't count." But after all this time, in which many different forms of birth control have become available, unwanted pregnancies are still highly prevalent in this country. What this tells us is that despite the information and products available for birth control, we as a culture are still behaving irresponsibly. Is there any excuse for this neglect?

In today's lexicon, "safer sex" is often associated with HIV and AIDS. There is no question that AIDS (acquired immune deficiency syndrome) deserves every bit of the attention it has received. This disease not only kills, but often strips people of all their hope, dignity, and quality of life. Happily, several advances have been made in medicine that allow persons infected with HIV to live longer and healthier lives. However, since positive response to treatment is not a guarantee, prevention is a lot more effective.

That said, even if you are not in a high-risk group for HIV or AIDS, you may still be susceptible to infection. I asked Dr. Eric Daar, an immune disorders and AIDS specialist at Cedars-Sinai in Los Angeles, about men being infected with HIV by women, and he said, "I am currently treating a young man whose only risk factor was unprotected sex with a woman." The woman his patient slept with was not a prostitute. Dr. Daar then went on to discuss the thousands of women unwittingly infecting men in Africa and Asia, where HIV infection and AIDS exist mainly in the heterosexual, not homosexual, population.

The Numbers

The sheer number of men and women who have or have had one or more sexually transmitted diseases is quite astounding. One in every fifteen Americans will contract a sexually transmitted disease this year, and one in four Americans already has one. I cannot stress enough the importance of knowing whom you are sleeping with.

As I mentioned, many STDs have no obvious symptoms. For women, often the only time they become aware of an infection is when they take steps to start a family, and by then, the damage has already been done: A sleeping STD has robbed them of their ability to conceive a child. (Admittedly, sometimes the damage can be addressed and a woman can get pregnant through reproductive technologies, such as in vitro.)

Unfortunately, the lack of knowledge about a disease does not prohibit one from passing it on to somebody else, and this lack of awareness can go both ways. Men, too, can be asymptomatic of an infection and pass it along to their partners. Therefore, it is as much your responsibility to get tested as it is your partners'. If you have sex with someone who is carrying a sexually transmitted disease, you can get it, too. No one is immune from acquiring a sexually transmitted disease. Your age, race, ethnicity, or socioeconomic status will not protect you. The best agent of protection is yourself, so it's up to you to know the information, to be aware and considerate, and to take the time to ensure the safety of both of you.

Transmission

STDs can be spread through vaginal, oral, and anal sex. Some can also be spread through *any* contact between the penis and vulvar area, mouth, and/or anus. Sexually transmitted diseases can be spread from man to woman, woman to man, man to man, and woman to woman. Several STDs can be spread from mother to child at birth or through breast milk. And, as you are probably already aware, sharing needles can spread STDs, including HIV.

There is really only one way to be 100 percent sure you don't get a sexually transmitted disease: remain abstinent. But I think most of us (I'm including both men and women here) would feel a bit constrained if we gave up sex. The next less risky way to be sexual is to use your hands. Don't shrug off the fun you can have with your (or her) hands. You might be very surprised and eager to explore this territory of sexual delight. Make sure that your hands have no open wounds, abrasions, or cracked skin. Herpes and HPV, however, can be transmitted from genitals to hands (see below for more specific information on herpes and HPV). If you or your partner have either of these two viruses, you can protect yourselves by using latex gloves.

It's also true that genital-to-genital contact *without* intercourse can transmit some STDs, such as herpes and syphilitic lesions. The same is true during foreplay, in which any genital contact *at all* without condoms can be a problem. However, sometimes herpes is not restricted to the genitals and can manifest at the end of a nerve ganglion on the thigh or buttocks. Meeting that gorgeous stranger on the plane and inviting her for a few adult beverages, which you then follow with falling into the hotel bed, arms and legs in heated disarray, may not be the smartest move in this day and age. Instead, should you find yourself lusting after someone you just met, and both of you don't want to stop the inevitable, take a moment to talk about safer sex. I promise you, she will be grateful, and if not, you should be grateful you took care of you.

Responsible adults talk about sex beforehand. And after exchanging information with your new lover, use a condom. Until you've both tested negative for *all* sexually transmitted diseases and waited the appropriate incubation period to ensure a clean bill of health (without engaging in any risk behaviors in the meantime), you should continue to use condoms every single time you engage in vaginal, oral, or anal sex. As I am sure you're aware, condoms are available everywhere, in all sizes, styles, colors, and textures (there is a bounty of information on condoms at the end of this chapter).

For those of you roving males, you may not want to hear this, and I apologize in advance for sounding like your mother, but you can also reduce the risk of contracting an STD by limiting your number of sexual partners. The facts are plain: You are more likely to get a sexually transmitted disease if either of you has more than one partner at a time or if either of you has had a lot of previous partners. That's why the value of trust should never go underestimated in a relationship. What is often brushed aside or chalked up as one little indiscretion could have very serious health side effects. It's your choice, but I suggest being safe rather than sorry. Is one night of passion worth a lifetime of having lesions break out on your penis every month—or worse?

The Diseases

The following is a list of the most common sexually transmitted diseases along with their symptoms, potential dangers, and treatments and/or cures. This list is for your general information. It is not wise, under any circumstances, to self-diagnose when it comes to personal health. Several of these symptoms can be caused by factors other than an STD, and as I said earlier, many STDs can exist for a very long time before any symptoms are noticeable. If you think you have an STD, see your doctor.

If your physician confirms your suspicions, follow the medication instructions with accuracy, and tell your partner or partners immediately. There is no question that breaking the news can be difficult and awkward. But she needs to know for her own health in order to get treated, and so she doesn't potentially reinfect you. For more information about these and other sexually transmitted diseases, you can call the National STD Hotline at 800-227-8922 (see end of this chapter for further resources).

CHLAMYDIA

Chlamydia is caused by a bacterium that is also a parasite, meaning it needs other cells to exist and survive. It is often called the silent STD because there are usually no symptoms until the disease is in an advanced state. Men's symptoms include burning during urination, due to infection in the urethra, and epididymitis, inflammation and swelling of the epididymis on the testicles. By the late 1980s chlamydia had become the most common sexually transmitted bacterial infection in both North America and Europe. In 1997 the CDC reported 526,653 cases and estimates there are currently 3 million new occurrences annually. And 40 percent of nongonococcal urethritis (NGU) in men is caused by *Chlamydia trachomatis.*

SECRET FROM LOU'S ARCHIVES
Epididymitis, as a result of chlamydial infection, can lead to male infertility.

Chlamydia is spread through oral sex and intercourse. In women it can cause a bacterial infection deep within the fallopian tubes, causing chronic pain, tubal pregnancies, and/or infertility. With oral transmission, chlamydia can give you an upper respiratory infection. It can also be passed from mother to child during birth, causing eye, ear, and lung infections in newborns. The good news is that chlamydia is easily cured with antibiotics, but it must be tested for specifically.

GONORRHEA

Also referred to as the clap, gonorrhea is often associated with another century. However, the disease is still rampant in our country today. An estimated 600,000 new cases of gonorrhea will be contracted in the United States this year. Similar to chlamydia, it is a bacterial infection that can be completely asymptomatic. In women it often goes undetected until permanent damage has already occurred, including sterility, tubal pregnancies, and chronic pain. However, in men the symptoms can include a yellow puslike discharge from the penis, pain while urinating, the need to urinate often, and pain in the lower abdomen. This STD is highly contagious and can be spread through any contact with the penis, vulvar area, mouth, or anus, even without penetration.

The good news is that if detected early, gonorrhea is easily curable with antibiotics.

SYPHILIS

Syphilis is a very dangerous bacterial infection, and an estimated 104,000 new cases in men and women will be contracted in the United States this year. If left untreated, syphilis can be fatal and/or cause irreparable damage to the heart, brain, eyes, and joints. Forty percent of all babies born to mothers with syphilis die during childbirth or are born with abnormal features. Symptoms are painless sores, rash on the palms and feet, and swollen lymph nodes. This disease is highly contagious through oral, vaginal, and anal sex, as well as through open wounds on the skin. When detected early, syphilis is curable with strong doses of antibiotics. Syphilis is common in heterosexual men in certain parts of the country and very rare in others.

HERPES

What is most startling about genital herpes is how widespread it is among the American population. It is estimated that somewhere between 200,000 and 500,000 new cases of genital herpes will be contracted this year and that 45 million Americans are infected already. Even more frightening is the number of people who are not aware of already being infected.

There are two viruses that cause genital herpes: herpes simplex 1, which occurs orally, and herpes simplex 2, which occurs genitally. Herpes simplex 1 is typically what we refer to as cold sores on, around, or inside the lips and mouth. The visible symptoms of herpes simplex 2 include itchy bumps or tiny blisters on the genital area of men, typically on the shaft of the penis, at the end of the foreskin, or near the head of the penis. In women the outbreak occurs near or inside the vagina and labia or rectum. Men can also get herpes near the anus even if they have never had anal intercourse. Sometimes herpes lesions first appear in areas related to the genitals by nerve endings but not actually on the genitals. In this case, the buttocks and thighs are common.

SECRET FROM LOU'S ARCHIVES

If you or your lady has active cold sores, do not receive or give oral sex, as you can transmit herpes simplex 1 genitally.

It is a common myth that herpes lesions always cause great pain. Usually, it is pressure on a herpes sore that makes it hurt. Herpes can be contracted on any area of skin or mucous membrane, depending upon what area was in intimate contact with a lesion. The first outbreak of genital herpes may last between twelve and fourteen days, and is typically the most severe, while subsequent outbreaks are shorter in duration (four to five days) and milder. However, nowadays most people with herpes never get this first bad episode and just start out with mild or asymptomatic infection.

Herpes is highly contagious when physical contact is made during an outbreak, but it can also be contagious when the virus appears to lie dormant. This is because it can reactivate without symptoms in most people with herpes. Lab studies have found that in cases in which a person feels that herpes is not active, 5 percent of the time evidence of the infectious virus can be found on the skin.

The key to remember is to get any localized change or inflammation of the skin or blister or chafed area checked out while you can still see it. However, if you think you have been exposed to herpes, there is only one test, a blood test called the Western blot, that can make this diagnosis without symptoms. Doctors more often perform viral culture tests by swabbing a lesion when it is in a very early stage of blistering or erosions.

I understand that it is awkward and difficult to tell your partner that you are infected, especially in a new relationship. As one man, a math professor from Los Angeles, told me, "I had met this terrific woman and I was terrified to tell her I had herpes. I remember lying in bed with her; we hadn't done anything at this point, and I knew I had to tell her. I was afraid that once she knew, she wouldn't want to continue the relationship. When I told her, she wasn't pleased to hear the news, but I told her that I had got it from a woman who hadn't known she was infected. We didn't have sex that night. After a day, she came back to me and said that she did want to continue our relationship and that it was how I told her the news that made the difference. I was thrilled."

There is no cure for this virus, though the oral medications acyclovir, famciclovir, and valacyclovir have proved to be highly successful in both minimizing the symptoms of current outbreaks and suppressing recurrences. Furthermore, these agents will reduce the rate of asymptomatic shedding, and studies are under way to determine if this can reduce transmission, too.

What, precisely, determines a herpes recurrence has not been determined. Studies indicate there is a strong association between herpes outbreaks and sun and stress. Yet in and of itself, herpes can be stressful—both physically (it can be tiring) and emotionally. As one seminar attendee said, "When I found out I had herpes, I felt like a complete leper. I was furious at the guy who gave it to me and have been celibate ever since. I wouldn't ever want anyone to have to go through this hell." But others take the information in stride: "After we'd had our AIDS tests and knew we were going to sleep together, she told me she had herpes. I was pretty sure we were both okay HIV-wise but this came out of left field. I won't deny it made me think twice, but she has always been hypercareful about anything, so we invariably use condoms."

While the symptoms of herpes virus can be uncomfortable to those who have them, another real danger of this sexually transmitted disease is to an unborn child or immune-suppressed individual with HIV or AIDS, for example. Newborn (neonatal) herpes is also a worry, but recent information shows that this is very unlikely in cases where the mother has herpes before pregnancy. It is most often transmitted during delivery and can cause painful blisters and damage to the eyes, brain, and internal organs of a newborn baby. One in six newborns will not survive at all.

The good news is that when knowledge of genital herpes exists, a cesarean delivery can generally prevent damage to the child. In fact, the risk is so low these days that women who are having recurrent herpes are only given a cesarean section if there is an active symptomatic lesion present. However, the important point about neonatal herpes is that it is caused by men. The woman at greatest risk for having an affected baby experiences her transmission and first episode late in pregnancy. Therefore, if you and your partner are working on getting pregnant, and you have herpes and your partner does not, it is paramount for you to use proper safer sex practices during the pregnancy and consider suppressive antiviral treatment.

HPV

The human papilloma virus, also known as condyloma, represents a family of viruses that consists of more than eighty different types. There will be an estimated 1 million new cases of HPV diagnosed this year. Certain forms of HPV cause visible genital warts, though some strains cause no warts at all. Genital warts are growths that appear on the penis, scrotum, groin, or thigh. They can be raised or flat, single or multiple, small or large. All sexually active men and women are susceptible to contracting HPV. It is spread by direct contact during vaginal, oral, or anal sex with someone who has the virus. In women they can be on the external or internal genitals, and though rare, infants can be infected during childbirth.

SECRET FROM LOU'S ARCHIVES

In the Seattle study of eighteen-year-olds, 25 percent of girls who had been sexually active for one year had already been infected with HPV.

Because HPV is a virus that can lie dormant for years, you may suddenly have an outbreak after being monogamous for years. The diagnosis of HPV is usually made clinically, based on appearance. Special tests for the virus are available but are not generally done when you go to the doctor for a clean bill of health. No effective blood test is yet available, but scientists are working on one. In the meantime, since there is no known cure for this disease, I suggest limiting partners and using safer sex. Men need to check themselves regularly, as they do for any signs of testicular abnormalities, for example. You should also encourage the woman in your life to get Pap smears regularly, and look for any new growths on the skin, which even if painless, should be checked out. Infectiousness correlates to some extent with the appearance and disappearance of the actual lesions.

It is important to know that the majority of people who acquire a strain of the virus never develop a disease. However, there are five common types of HPV that are associated with cervical cancer. The strains that cause genital warts, though, are not the same strains associated with cervical cancer. While cancer is a rare consequence in men, some women are plagued by irritating warts and/or show abnormal Pap smears. Besides being painful, certain strains of HPV can cause cervical abnormalities, which can be cancerous. Only the physician can sort this out. Genital warts can be treated in several ways, including freezing, laser surgery, and topical creams. Some are applied by the doctor and some by the person with warts. None are cures. The strains of HPV that don't produce genital warts usually go undetected until a woman has an abnormality in her Pap smear. Genital HPV is manageable with proper diagnosis.

HEPATITIS B

Infection caused by the hepatitis B virus is not usually considered an STD; however, it is spread through infected semen, vaginal secretions, and saliva, and it is one hundred times more infectious than HIV. You can get hepatitis B from vaginal, oral, or—especially— anal sex. You can also get infected with the virus through direct contact with an infected person via open sores or cuts. This means that if someone in your home is infected, you can contract hepatitis B by using the same razor or toothbrush.

Hepatitis B attacks the liver. In its mildest form, you may never know you have it, but some carriers develop cirrhosis and/or liver cancer. Your chances of contracting liver cancer are two hundred times higher if you're a carrier of hepatitis B. Symptoms, when they appear, can be very much like those of the stomach flu. See your doctor immediately if you have nausea, unexplainable tiredness, dark urine, and/or yellowing of the eyes and skin. New effective and safe treatments are now available. However, the vast majority of people who get hepatitis B as adults recover all on their own.

There is a vaccination for hepatitis B. It is a series of shots, given in the arm. You must have all three shots to be safe. (The hepatitis A vaccination is a two-shot series, not three.) If you know your partner has hepatitis B, the vaccine will protect you after you have completed the shots, but you should have a test to make sure you responded. People with no special known risk (such as an infected partner) probably do not need the test—just the shots. This is the only STD vaccine that works and it is widely available.

Hepatitis B mainly attacks young men and women in their teens and twenties, and once you contract it, you have a small chance of becoming a carrier for life or even getting chronic liver problems or cancer. This year in the United States, there will be between 140,000 and 320,000 new cases of hepatitis B documented. Not all doctors and nurses are aware of this fast-growing problem in their communities, so don't hesitate to ask for your vaccination—especially if you are someone who is changing partners frequently. Hepatitis B is easily passed from mother to unborn child. It is also transmissible to young children and infants, but can be largely prevented by vaccination of infants at birth.

HIV / AIDS

The expected number of people in the United States who will contract HIV this year is 45,000, and the number of new infections is not yet declining. The chilling part of this statistic is that even though we know how to prevent HIV transmission and have aggressive new antiviral therapies to deal with it, we are not taking the most important step: preventing the spread of it.

Centers for Disease Control (CDC) figures documented in February 1999 show that in the United States the majority (51 percent) of HIV-infected individuals are heterosexual. Does this get your attention, gentlemen? I hope so. I don't mean to use scare tactics here, but I do feel obligated to give you the real information. In addition, the average age of those becoming infected has become younger, with a marked increase in the number of infected adolescents.

HIV and AIDS are not the same thing. Unfortunately, one is the precursor of the other. Acquired immune deficiency syndrome (AIDS) is a diagnosis resulting from infection with a virus known as the human immunodeficiency virus (HIV). When someone tests positive for HIV, his or her system has been exposed to the virus and his/her body is presenting an immune response to it.

You cannot get AIDS without having the human immunodeficiency virus. You can, however, be HIV positive without having an AIDS diagnosis. HIV attacks the immune system, leaving the body unable to fight off common sicknesses or other diseases. It is a sexually infectious disease spread through bodily fluids that are high in white blood cells: blood, semen, vaginal fluids, and mother's breast milk. It is not an airborne virus and cannot be spread by casual contact. Touching, food, coughs, mosquitoes, toilet seats, swimming in pools, and donating blood do *not* spread HIV. Transmission is not through saliva. In very rare cases, HIV has been known to be transmitted from a highly infected person through kissing or biting, resulting from poor oral hygiene from open bleeding gums or mouth sores. It is the high vascularization (i.e., a lot of blood supply close to the surface) of mucosal tissues of the anus, mouth, and vagina that makes these areas the most vulnerable to infection.

There are usually no symptoms accompanying HIV. People can get the virus and feel terrific for many years. A small percentage of people will develop an acute mononucleosis-like illness during primary infection. Left untreated, the virus almost always leads to

AIDS, and because it is the immune system that fails, the symptoms for AIDS can look like anything from a cold to cancer.

Although there is no cure for AIDS, there are new drugs that dramatically slow down the effect that HIV has on the immune system. It can take up to six months for one's immune system to show antibodies, which means that you have tested positive for exposure. Every sexually active man and woman should have two HIV tests—one after risky behavior and another after waiting six months. The six-month waiting period will ensure a clean bill of health before having unprotected sex with any new partner. Sadly, in this day and age, it isn't always enough to accept a verbal declaration of good health. Many, many people have been deceived by lovers who claimed to be HIV negative and weren't.

In one reported case, a young mother didn't realize she was infected with HIV until her daughter was born. When her physician gave her the terrible news, she was shocked. Immediately, she and her husband were tested and both were found HIV positive. As you can imagine, each suspected the other of not having been truthful about a past experience. It turned out that before they were married, the husband had had a fling with an old girlfriend. Since the two knew each other well, neither bothered to use safer sex (she was on the pill). Unfortunately, the woman didn't know she had been infected and unwittingly passed it on to the man, creating a domino effect of infection.

It is very important that you ask to see the results of your lover's HIV test and all tests for sexually transmitted diseases, especially in the case of (but not limited to) women you don't know well (consider going together to get tested). It is also important that she see the results of yours. In fact, rather than make her ask to see yours, offer your results as a show of good faith, opening the door for her to do the same. If your lover refuses to show you her test results, it may be wise to refuse to have unprotected sex with her. Remember, she is being secretive about something that affects *your* health and quite possibly your life. No one should want to keep her/his good health a secret.

When obtaining an HIV test, be mindful of the difference between confidential and anonymous testing. They are not the same. When you have an *anonymous test*, you are identified by a number or letter only, not by your name, your Social Security number, or any other identifying information. After the blood sample is taken, you confirm that the numbers/letters on the vial and the numbers/letters on your identification slip are the same. A week later you go back to the clinic where the test was taken and get the results. Typically, no results are given over the phone. A *confidential test* means that the results are confidential and limited only by the integrity of those who have access to the information. In other words, you are using your name and placing your trust in the doctor, nurse, or clinic where you get tested. Two years ago an employee at a southern clinic copied the names of all those who had tested positive for HIV and sold the list for fifty dollars a page at a local bar. Clearly, this was a completely unethical act by an amoral person, and it is not commonplace. You can never be 100 percent sure with confidential testing, however, and may be better off with anonymous testing.

There is a new method of testing for HIV, called Orasure, an oral specimen collection device that requires no blood collection and is 99 percent accurate. Like a blood test it too tests for the presence of HIV antibodies. Dr. Penelope Hitchcock says that Orasure is a great product and that the NIH are now working with the manufacturer.

In certain populations there has been a marked growth in infections. For example, the senior women population in South Florida has shown recent growth. Dr. Eric Daar points out that the infection figures have grown because this population wasn't really aware of the health or risk issues regarding HIV, AIDS, and other STDs. Consequently, these women and men are getting infected because they are not using protection. Since the women aren't worried about pregnancy, they figure they have no need for that stuff at their age. By assuming that their partners are all okay, they have put themselves in danger of infection. As I noted above, there is also a marked increase in infections among adolescents. This group is particularly vulnerable because sometimes they are not as open to listening or paying attention to safe sex information.

Finally, I'd like to make several important points about HIV/AIDS:

Point #1: There are several clades (or types) of the HIV virus: A, B, C, D, E, F, M, and O. And within each clade there are different strains. So even if a man or a woman is already positive, he or she can still become infected by another form of virus and is even more susceptible, given the already weakened state of the immune system.

Point #2: The most common clade in North America and Europe is B, and for Southeast Asia it is E. Central Africa is a melting pot of different clades.

Point #3: Some strains appear to be more virulent than others. Depending on the virulence of the strain one is exposed to, you could have an almost immediate AIDS diagnosis.

Point #4: "HIV positive" means you have been exposed to the virus that causes AIDS. Your body shows a positive immune response to HIV.

Point #5: In 1993 the CDC created a definition benchmark for an AIDS diagnosis. This enabled physicians to diagnose AIDS in a uniform manner and also better qualify people for health insurance coverage and drug programs.

Point #6: It is suggested that you wait six months after risky behavior before getting tested. This is because it can take up to six months for antibodies to show up in a test, although most people (95 percent) test positive within three months of exposure, using the antibodies testing methods.

Point #7: A test called a PCR (Polymerase Chain Reaction) tests for the actual virus in your blood. Estimate that someone who is going to seroconvert (go from HIV– to HIV+) can start to have the virus in his or her system within five to seven days of exposure; on average it takes two weeks for seroconversion. This is an expensive test. It is not an accepted screening test but is occasionally used by groups at very high risk, such as pornography actors.

Point #8: Four years ago there was hope that with the powerful antiviral medications that had HIV+ people walking around with little to no detectable viral load, they would be able to stop therapy at some point. That no longer appears to be the case, as there seem to be reservoirs of HIV in the body. Still, there is a small amount of hope that even more treatments might clear the virus completely in some people in the future. Right now, these treatments are just experimental. The better we get at detecting the virus in the laboratory, the better we are at successfully treating those who are infected.

Point #9: Just because someone has no detectable viral load does not mean he or she cannot infect someone else.

Point #10: In 1998 the CDC estimated that 80 percent of people who are HIV+ do not know they are infected because they have never been tested.

Point #11: An opportunistic infection is one that would not be a threat to a healthy, normal immune system but takes the "opportunity" to attack a compromised immune system. For example, a person who is undergoing cancer treatment such as chemotherapy is at risk for an opportunistic infection. Every infection, however, isn't an opportunistic one.

While I've discussed the most common of the sexually transmitted diseases, there are more than fifty known STDs to date. Providing you with knowledge about them is not meant to scare you, but rather to empower you. No one should have to be frightened into taking control of his sexual health. Rather, with this information, I hope being safe and careful becomes a matter of self-respect. Without protection, there just isn't an excuse good enough to participate in a sexual relationship with someone whose health you're not 100 percent sure about. You don't drive without car insurance. You don't go through life without health or home insurance. The same applies to sexual safety. It's absolutely your responsibility to be honest about your health status and communicate this to your partner, no matter how casual or close your relationship. It's also your responsibility to make sure you are not unwittingly passing a disease on to a lover.

Choosing a Condom

There are many different condoms to choose from, but not all of them are made with quality. The chart below can give you the wide range of styles, sizes, textures, and other features of condoms. However, before purchasing, you may want to consider the following information.

> ➤ Condoms break. Any condom can break during intercourse,
> for many different reasons. Breakage is almost invariably the
> result of improper handling, such as using teeth to open the
> foil or keeping condoms in wallets or car glove boxes, where

heat will eventually break down the latex in the condom, making it easier to burst. Any lubricant with an oil or petroleum base (e.g., Vaseline) will also break down and destroy latex condoms. Also, the compressed rectangular packaging of some condom brands reduces the longevity of the condoms themselves.

➤ During a study conducted by Dr. Bruce Voeller, founder of the Mariposa Foundation, men who were chronic condom "busters" were discovered to have been using everyday hand lotion as a lubricant. A lubricant must be water-based, and most hand lotions contain some form of oil. Oil is a latex condom's mortal enemy because it immediately begins to erode the latex. Therefore, it is imperative that the ingredients of a lotion be checked carefully before using with a latex condom. Better still, use a water-based lubricant intended for this purpose, such as Astroglide, Sensura, or Liquid Silk. (There is more complete information on lubrication in Chapter Five.)

➤ The most often heard excuse from men who have had unprotected sex is that they don't like condoms because they diminish the pleasure factor. That isn't the question here: It's a matter of safety. However, after you both have been tested and waited the six-month period to make sure you're both healthy, during which you have had no risk factors or sex with anyone else, and then are tested a second time, you will be free and clear to use other methods of birth control.

➤ One of the excuses I hear from men in my seminars is that they are too big to fit into any of the condoms currently available. In my seminars, I usually open a regular-size condom, shape my fingers into a bird's beak, and, watching my nails, unroll the condom over my hand and stretch/pull it down so that it covers my entire forearm past my elbow (it fits, trust me). How much bigger can you be than that? Try it yourself if you don't believe me.

➤ For those gentlemen who have thick, broad penises, there are condoms specifically manufactured with this in mind. These men find regular condoms fit a little too snugly at the base of the shaft and/or at the head. There are two large-size condoms available, Magnum and Trojan-Enz. Field researchers definitely prefer the Magnum. They say the Trojans smell awful and have a "yucky" texture. There is also a larger-head condom coming back onto the market under the name Pleasure Plus. This condom has a baggier head that allows for more friction and stimulation and is completely different in sensation. A similar sensation can be achieved with a regular condom by putting a jelly-bean size dollop of lubricant into the end of the condom before putting it on.

> ### SECRET FROM LOU'S ARCHIVES
> Because the herpes and human papilloma viruses can affect skin not covered by a condom, the efficiency of condoms is not as good as it might be for HIV or chlamydia, which are generally contracted from body fluids. However, you can add to your protection if you avoid contact when lesions are active and use condoms religiously at other times.

➤ As the only manufactured spermicidal in the United States, nonoxynol-9 was introduced into the United States in 1920 as a cleaning solution in hospitals. This very irritating substance is found in any diaphragm gel, contraceptive foam, contraceptive sheets, cervical caps, or condoms that contain spermicide. As a spermicidal (i.e., it kills sperm), it breaks down the lipid (fat) layer of the sperm. If it sears this outer layer of sperm, can you imagine what it does to the surface of *her* skin? On contact, this substance can literally burn her. Imagine taking detergent and rubbing it on the most delicate area of the woman you love. I have also heard from many women who have been exposed to nonoxynol-9 that they have experienced constant bladder and vaginal infections. If you or she is experiencing any irritation, you may want to avoid this nasty substance. As one seminar attendee told me, "My wife and I started using a diaphragm with foam after our son was born a year ago. She had constant vaginal infections, which never seemed to go away. She was in constant pain, and we eventually stopped having sex. Sure enough, when I learned from your seminar about nonoxynol-9, we discovered that had been the culprit. Within a week of our stopping using the foam, everything cleared up." In addition, nonoxynol-9 reduces the average five-year shelf life of condoms by two years.

➤ Although you may hear differently, spermicides containing nonoxynol-9 were created to help reduce the risk of unwanted pregnancy, *not* sexually transmitted diseases. Nonoxynol-9 has proved to be effective at killing *only* HIV and herpes in laboratory tests. There are *no* studies showing nonoxynol-9 has a risk-free effect on human beings. There are *no* studies showing it interferes with the transmission of HIV in normal activity. It has been shown to kill HIV and STDs in test tubes, but there is no clinical evidence to suggest it is a safe measure for disease prevention.

➤ There is long-term research under way for other microbicidal products, but they are not near completion. According to Dr. Penelope Hitchcock, Chief of Sexually Transmitted Diseases Bureau of the National Institutes of Health, the best protection against HIV, gonorrhea, and pregnancy is the male latex condom used properly and correctly every time one has sex. But keep in mind that 10 percent of the population is allergic to latex.

> **SECRET FROM LOU'S ARCHIVES**
>
> "My fiancée used to use those contraceptive sheets, the kind that are inserted like a tampon. Well, I started to get this awful burning sensation in my penis in the middle of sex. Finally, I figured out it was the contraceptive sheet with nonoxynol-9 that was getting rammed into the end of my penis. I would be sore for days and peeing was really painful."

➤ Spermicides should be used only in addition to condoms, never in place of them.

➤ Beware of condoms labeled as "novelty" condoms, such as "glow-in-the-dark." These are not intended to provide pregnancy or STD protection.

➤ The "ribbed for her pleasure" condoms do nothing for women. They were designed so men would buy them thinking they did something—they don't.

➤ French ticklers are best for their laugh factor, not the pleasure factor. Why? Because up at the nether reaches of

CONDOM BRANDS	Box Desc. Lubrication (At time of publication.)**	Size in mm (Metric) ##	Condom Features 1. Thickness 2. Surface Feel 3. Slim/Wide Fit 4. Size Variation
LATEX			
Kimono Microthin	Dark Blue Silicone	170 x 49 mm	1. Ultra Thin 3. Slimmer
Trojan-Enz Lubricated	??? Silicone	185 x 52 mm	4. Oversized available in Green box
Paradise Super Sensitive	White/Black Silicone	180 x 52 mm	1. Ultra Thin and Pinky Sheer
Crown Skin Less Skin	White/Blue Silicone	180 x 55 mm	1. Ultra Thin 3. Slimmer
Contempo Exotica	Blue/Woman Silicone	180 x 49 mm	3. Slim Fitting
Vis-a-Vis Ultra Thin	Multi-Colored Silicone	165 x 49 mm	1. Ultra Thin
Trojan Ultra Thin	Grey Silicone	185 x 52 mm	4. Baggy Shape for greater friction
LifeStyles Ultra Sensitive	Light Grey Silicone	180 x 52 mm	1. Ultra Thin
InVigra	Royal Blue Silicone	185 x 52 mm	1. Regular
Contempo Wet n' Wild	Woman/Thong Silicone	180 x 52 mm	2. Generous Lubrication
Paradise Extra Large	Black/Purple	190 x 56 mm	3. Wider Fit
Magnum	Black/gold Silicone	180 x 56 mm	3. Wider Fit
Pleasure Plus	Metallized Silicon	175 x 52 mm	4. Oversized end & slight ribbing heightens sensation
Lifestyle Discs.	Individual Blister Pack	4. Separate pack per condom	
NATURAL			
Naturalamb Skin Kling Tite	Black Jelly-Type	165 x 55 mm	Most natural feel
POLYURETHANE			
Avanti for Men	Black with Swirl Silicone	N/A	United Kingdom
Supra	Gold Silicone		N/A
Reality for Women	Pouch Silicone	175 mm—7"	N/A
FLAVORED			
Kiss of Mint	Green Non lubricated	180 x 52 mm	Real flavor not just fragrance

Most popular condom for Nevada legal prostitution establishments: Contempo Bareback with no nonoxynol-9. They will be switching to Invigra Fall of '99. Best-seller in grocery stores: Trojans. and Best-seller in Adult Stores: Contempo RoughRider. (The name sells it as the little bumps do nothing for the lady.)

Country of Manufacture Distributor	Average Retail Cost	Where to Purchase: Drugstore, Supermarket, MailOrder, Internet, Adult Novelty Store	Field Researchers Comments & F.Y.I.
Japan Mayer Labs	$11 for 12	D/S/M/I/A	Light and strong
USA Carter-Wallace	$8-10 for 12	D/S/M/I/A	Leading condom in sales at retail
India Paradise Marketing	$7-9 for 12	D/S/M/I/A	Similar to Crown condoms
Japan Okamoto-USA	$8-10 for 12	D/S/M/I/A	So sheer and invisible used in porn films
Thailand Ansel	$7-9 for 12	M/I/A	Nice and snug for the slimmer man
Japan Sagami	$7-9 for 12	D/S/M/I/A	Really sheer
US Carter-Wallace	$8-10 for 12	D/S/M/I/A	Known name
Thailand Ansel	$7-9 for 12	D/S/M/I/A	Identical Condom to Comtempo Bareback
India Paradise Marketing	$6-7 for 12	D/S/M/I/A	Similar to Lifestyle Lub., & Trojan-Enz Lub., but less $
Thailand Ansel	$7-9 for 12	M/I/A	Lifestyles Lubricated Identical Condom
Malaysia Paradise Marketing	$8-10 for 12	D/S/M/I/A	New larger style available Fall of '99
USA Carter-Wallace	$9-10 for 12	D/S/M/I/A	Best for Italian Method Sheerest of larger condoms
China Global	$16-20 for 12	D/S/M/I/A	Similar to InSpiral & LifeStyles Extra Pleasure
	$8 for 6	D/S/M/I/A	Clear instructions
USA Carter-Wallace	$9-10 for 3	D/S/M/I/A	Great pregnancy protection if not concerned about STDs
	$8-9 for 3 Durex/L.I.H.	D/S/M/I/A	Too much breakage
USA Trojan-Carter-Wallace	$6-7 for 3	D/S/M/I/A with nonoxynol-9	Available ONLY with nonoxynol-9
Britain Female Health Co.	$2-3 for 1	D/S/M/I/A	Protection women can control
Thailand Ansel	$7-9 for 12	D/S/M/I/A	Best of all the "flavored" condoms

** All latex condom packages describe those WITHOUT nonoxynol-9. All male latex condoms available with or without nonoxynol-9.
\#\# Condom widths—49 mm slim fit. 52 mm average width. 56 mm wider fit.

the vaginal barrel most women only have an awareness of pressure sensation, not little hats on condoms.

➤ If you're shy about purchasing condoms, there are several mail-order catalogs available. See the resource section at the end of Chapter Seven.

➤ There is a male polyurethane condom on the market (Avanti), which states on its label that it has not been tested for protection; I recommend staying away from this brand until its product testing is done. Trojan is coming out with a new polyurethane product, Supra, but will only be available with nonoxynol-9.

➤ As of June 1999 the major manufacturers of condoms in the United States, Ansell and Carter-Wallace, had pretty much shut down domestic production and are now having product manufactured in offshore plants. The plants here were old, with dated equipment from the 1960s and 1980s, which wasn't adaptable to the needs of the contemporary market. Ansell makes Lifestyles, Contempo, Prime; Carter-Wallace makes Trojans, Class Act, and Magnums.

SECRET FROM LOU'S ARCHIVES

The FDA allowable failure rate for condoms is 4 in 1,000 picked randomly.

Techniques for Safe Sex

Putting on a condom doesn't have to interrupt the momentum or excitement of your sexual experience; instead, by sharing the procedure with your partner, you can actually increase the play or erotic factor. Let her put the condom on you, for instance, or put it on together, using both your hands to roll it down. For the more adventurous women, there is the Italian Method, which was illustrated in my previous book. This method involves the woman putting a condom on using her mouth.

Another fun trick to try is placing a dollop of condom-safe (water-soluble, latex-safe) lubricant the size of a jelly bean in the nipple end of the condom before you put it on. This will enhance the sensation for you by reducing that "stuck on" feeling.

Resources

Safety is essential, but it doesn't have to undermine the sensuality of your lovemaking. Being aware of the risks and taking preventive measures will only increase your connection with your partner and maintain the honesty of your relationship. The following is a list of resources you can contact for further information.

FREE INFORMATION AND REFERRALS ABOUT SEXUALLY TRANSMITTED DISEASES (STDs)

Centers for Disease Control
Website: www.cdc.gov
Public Health Service AIDS Hotline
800-342-AIDS (24 hours a day, 7 days a week)

STD National Hotline (Centers for Disease Control)
800-227-8922 (8:00 A.M.–11:00 P.M. EST weekdays)
website: www.ashastd.org

Hepatitis Hotline (Centers for Disease Control)
888-443-7232
or American Liver Foundation
800-223-0179

National Herpes Hotline
919-361-8488

ABOUT SEXUALITY

American Association of Sex Educators, Counselors and Therapists
(AASECT)
P. O. Box 238
Mt. Vernon, Iowa 52314
www.AASECT.org
Can provide a list of AASECT-certified therapists in your area.

Society for the Scientific Study of Sexuality (aka the 4Ss)
www.sscwisc.edu/ssss

American Board of Sexology
email: billeast@ctinet.net
Can provide referrals to Diplomates and Clinical Supervisors
in your area.
Bill East is the executive director.
(202) 462-2122

Sex Information Education Council of the United States (SEICUS)
212-819-9770

———— • ————

THREE

Getting Her
in the Mood

The Two Rs

Most of us divide sex into two stages: foreplay followed by intercourse. As in most sports—tennis, for example—we usually spend
some time warming up, and then we feel ready for "the real game."
I'd like to turn that particular formula on its head. First, in order to
have great, fabulous, mind-blowing sex, you've got to have great, fabulous, mind-blowing foreplay. This is especially true for women, who
can barely enjoy intercourse without first having foreplay. So what
exactly is foreplay? For women, foreplay has two essential stages.
The first stage works on her brain, and the second works on her body.
In this chapter, I will show you how to seduce her mind. It's actually
quite simple: First you romance her and then you relax her.

These two steps are simple in concept, but I cannot overempha-
size how crucial they are to successfully getting her in the mood for
sex so she can truly let go and let you bring her to the heights of pleasure. Relaxing and romancing combine two of the most potent forms
of mental foreplay (we will discuss physical foreplay in Chapter

Five). The reason these two activities hold such sway is that they are controlled by our most powerful sexual organ—the brain.

Romance and Courtly Behavior

It has been my observation that the surest way to guarantee a man's ability to turn on a woman and drive her mad with desire is through good old-fashioned courting. I am absolutely serious, and this does not contradict all those voices in your head and hers saying that she wants to be treated as your equal partner. No woman wants to give up that mutuality. However, women do want to feel special and singular, and the best way you can make them feel special is by being a gentleman and treating her like a lady. After all, it is a very simple equation: Only a man can be a gentleman and treat a lady as a lady, and since there are fewer and fewer real gentlemen out there, those of you who adopt this courting policy will have a genuine market advantage.

In order to behave like a gentleman, you need to think like one. Again, it comes down to your attitude. If a woman feels you're being solicitous and caring, taking her pleasure and comfort into consideration, chances are she will hand you carte blanche. This is, of course, assuming you've already passed her litmus test.

One of the primary ingredients of courtly behavior is having good manners. Sadly, many parents no longer teach their young boys manners, and many men have just lost the habit even if they were taught early on in life. Yet manners, quite simply, are nothing other than pleasant and respectful ways of interacting with others.

What are good manners? Be polite, be courteous, and treat her as you know she wishes to be treated. There are certain social niceties that only a gentleman can perform. Please know this is not an exhaustive list but merely an outline, so feel free to add or subtract as you wish.

Open a door for a lady. This particular gesture often receives a bum rap, and yet for most women it is a lovely acknowledgment of how you think of her. Having said that, I must admit that I have had men tell me unpleasant tales of women sneering at them when they try this move. As a fully emancipated, independent woman, I find a woman's rejection of this masculine attempt at being courteous just plain sad. I love this social acknowledgment of my femininity and I believe that, deep down, most women will admit they enjoy being treated like a lady as well. Many men have also told me that they get pleasure from being courteous and wish only for a woman to smile or nod her head in appreciation.

The historic rationale for a lady entering a room before a gentleman was not so enchanting or courtly. Supposedly in less civilized, war-torn times, men would "toss" a woman through an unknown entry in order to test for enemies. Considered less valuable than men, women were quite literally sacrificial social lambs. This rationale then changed to women leading the entry of a man in order to introduce his wealth and status: The more beautiful and bejeweled the woman, the more important the man. In some social circles, this attitude may not have changed all that much.

Opening the car door. Have you heard the joke about being able to tell who the wife is by who has to climb the snowbank to get in the car? Suffice it to say that if you let the woman in your life know from the get-go that you'd like to open the car door for her, nine times out of ten, she will love and appreciate the gesture. If this is an entirely new ritual for you, it may take some time getting used to—for both of you—but I believe it may be a pleasant and rewarding courtly move to add to your growing repertoire. The mother of a male friend of mine from Louisiana will not get in or out of the car unless a man opens the door for her. This may be taking things to an extreme, but I give her credit for standing by what she believes in. If you have a low-slung car, you may want to offer your hand to help balance her as she gets in.

If the two of you are getting in or out of a cab, bus, or other public conveyance, you might also consider offering your hand or arm to help her alight.

Stand when a lady enters or leaves a room. Please note that this move is appropriate for social situations, not business. When I was in private school, we were expected to stand whenever a teacher entered or left the room. This was a very clear display of respect for our elders. However, in social situations, standing for a woman, even simply raising yourself from a chair, can be a wonderful gesture of consideration and civility. Men in the seminars have made comments such as "When I do something so simple, it makes such an impact on her. I know she knows I care about her."

Pull out her chair. Like parallel parking, this move takes awareness, several front and back moves, and finesse. If she is returning from the ladies' room, you don't need to jump to your feet. Instead, gently pull out or slide her chair as she returns to the table. She will be doing the majority of the work, so you need not jump up behind her like a butler.

Take her arm or place your hand on the small of her back. Both of these moves can be used publicly and socially, and they are the least objectionable PDAs (public displays of affection). Holding hands and draping your arm around her shoulders is more informal and therefore not suggested for public events. Rather, these moves are best saved for the weekend stroll, sitting in the movie theater, or at the table, where the intimacy is about the two of you.

Carry items for her. One woman related, "I remember my boyfriend telling me when we first met that he would carry all my packages when I went shopping. He didn't want me to carry anything but my purse. It took me a while to realize this was one of his unspoken ways to say 'I love you' and that he cares about me."

Then again, if a woman wants to carry her own bags, let her; it's her choice. But keep in mind that most women will welcome your wanting to help haul their belongings. Although carrying her shopping bags may be a broad-stroke example, choose another gesture that shows you are there for her, such as helping her into the house with the groceries or offering to move something heavy for her.

Have good table manners. Few things are a bigger turnoff than poor table manners. On the contrary, knowing how to behave at a table is very impressive to a woman and makes her feel she is with a man who knows what he's doing.

If the woman in your life likes strong fragrances, try tuberose, Casablanca, or Rubrum lilies. If these powerful flowers need a bit of toning down, add a spray of freesia, which is soft and gentle.

If you were never taught proper table manners, glance at an etiquette book in a book store.

Razzle-Dazzle Her

Beyond incorporating good manners into your courtly behavior, there are romantic ways to get her undivided attention. These suggestions are designed to take you and her one step closer to the intimacy of the bedroom.

Be the chef. More men are capturing a woman's heart with their culinary prowess. It happened to my identical twin sister. She felt airlifted when she first realized that among his many talents, her Greek husband is a wizard in the kitchen. Men who can cook are a huge turn-on. In the same way that a man feels loved and cared for when a woman cooks for him, a woman feels taken care of and oh so appreciated when a man cooks for her.

Breakfast in bed. If you prefer sex in the morning, breakfast in bed is a sure way to have her and yourself start out smiling and you will be her Prince Charming for a day—or at least the morning. You may want to avoid crunchy cereals such as granola. In this delicate position, it's better to err on the side of soft food, easily eaten with your fingers. Try pieces of fruit and soft Danishes or croissants that can be pulled apart easily. Prepare her coffee or tea just as she likes it—in front of her. This entails putting a small creamer and sugar or artificial-sweetener container on the tray. Let me suggest another tip: There are more interesting resting spots for that imported preserve than the English muffin she's nibbling on.

The art of flowers. Throughout the ages, gentlemen have presented flowers to their ladyloves as a sign of their feelings. Flowers are always a true gentleman's move, which make even more of an impact when you know her preferences. In other words, red roses are lovely and may be the first to come to mind, but often there is another flower that touches her heart more. One woman from a seminar shared this: "When my current boyfriend discovered I loved lavender, he checked out all the flower stands on the Upper West Side [of Manhattan] to find exactly what I liked. I didn't find out until his sister told me that he had hunted for two hours for them. You have to love a man who'll do that!" Another man told me, "If a guy sends a woman a dozen red roses after the first date, he either had a world-class date or he is not aware of the message he is sending. Red roses are not the casual thank-you flower."

SECRET FROM LOU'S ARCHIVES

Assuming you want the memory of you to last long, please send fresh-cut flowers. Preset arrangements and roses have the shortest life span of flowers. Arrangements are often the end buds of finishing flowers. And check the sepals of roses. These are the green "petals" at the base of the rosebud. If they are tight to the bud, it is a fresh rose. Otherwise you are getting old flowers that droop and will die in a day or two. Fresh roses should last five to seven days.

Relaxation Is Key

There is no getting around one simple fact: A typical woman will not get turned on if she isn't relaxed. That said, as a partner to this activity, you are being challenged to get her in the mood. How can you help her relax? You'll be happy (and perhaps relieved) to know that there are some tried-and-true ways to helping your partner loosen up so that she not only responds to you better but also enjoys herself more completely. As a forty-something physician told me, "I know I have to get my wife relaxed enough to get her turned on. If she can't relax, I know nothing is going to happen. And that's why I am king of foot massages." Another seminar attendee, an architect from Madison, Wisconsin, said that he draws his partner a hot bath, "with her favorite lavender salts. If she gets one whiff as she walks through the door, I know she's all mine."

But most men (and women) will agree that though the physical effects of your method are important, the key to relaxing her is *your* attitude. Quite simply, if she feels like you have gone out of your way to treat her as special, she will respond.

> **SECRET FROM LOU'S ARCHIVES**
> Relaxing can start twenty-four hours ahead of the game—in your head.

And why is relaxing so important for women? Because women's brains can juggle ten things at a time, and usually, out of necessity, they are doing just that. Unless the majority of those brain-juggling events are quieted, she won't be able to shift enough of her focus to the matters at hand. This is related to another one of those sex/gender differences: Women tend to experience their world in terms of relationships. Men tend to compartmentalize. In terms of sex, this means men can go into the bedroom and turn off whatever happened that day. Yet when women lie down, a steady stream of to-do lists can still be crossing the billboard of her mind. Therefore, gentlemen, you need to help her decompress and become still if you want to arouse her later. The connection is very concrete and very clear: Unless a woman is relaxed in her mind, her body will not follow suit. And if her body isn't relaxed, it won't get excited.

SECRET FROM LOU'S ARCHIVES

Did you know the word "negligee" suggests that the woman wearing it should relax and refrain from housework? It comes from the Latin *neglegere,* "to neglect," whose literal translation is "not to pick up."

IT'S ELEMENTARY

There are four essential elements to help a woman relax. Consider these in no particular order:

➤ Make her *comfortable*, mentally and physically.
➤ Minimize *interruptions*.
➤ Make the *space and time*, even if it is only ten minutes.
➤ Let her know you like *her body*.

1. Making her comfortable mentally and physically is about providing a good, safe, and enjoyable environment for a sexual encounter. For instance, if you are not married and do

not live together, try to make your bedroom a place that is inviting for her. Does she have a corner of the room, perhaps a drawer or a dresser where she can leave her toiletries or some clothes? If you are married or live together, make sure that you pay attention to the state of your bedroom as well, participating in keeping it tidy, putting away your clothes, or simply making sure the bed is made. One woman in a seminar shared this story: "I had just begun dating a man and we were getting serious. We'd already slept together, but never at his home. He was a very successful investment banker, who was always well groomed and wore nice clothes. But when I went to his apartment for the first time, I nearly died. It was filthy. The drapes were dirty, the shower curtain was moldy. I was disgusted and felt totally turned off. I made up some excuse that night and went home. A few days later I told him, in a nice way, that he needed to do something about his apartment. He had the money, after all. I think he just didn't know any better." Cleanliness is next to godliness in most women's eyes.

2. By minimizing interruptions, you keep the environment a haven for intimacy. This is why there are answering machines, locks on the doors, and for those of you who are parents, baby monitors. One woman explained, "We have a four-year-old and a nine-month-old. We both work and are typically exhausted at the end of the day. We plan an escape day away every month. We hire an overnight sitter and take off to a corporate suite or a friend's place who is away. This way we get to reconnect alone and rekindle what our romancing days were like when we were single. Then the problem was our crazy travel schedules, and we had to coordinate

months in advance to see one another. When we got married and the kids came, I initially felt guilty about leaving the kids. But the effect on our marriage has been miraculous! Two months ago our nine-month-old was sick and colicky, the four-year-old had just clogged the washing machine by pouring cat litter into it, and the gardener had flooded the storage area in the garage. We looked at one another amidst this chaos and both said at the same time, 'In two sleeps it will be Saturday,' which was our escape day. We both cracked up."

3. Make the space and time by planning. Just as you set aside time for your workout at the gym, a golf game, or a car tune-up, you need to set aside time for romance and relaxation. A woman from a seminar said that "the one thing that keeps me falling in love with my husband again and again is his ability to romance me. It can be something as simple as taking me into another room away from the kids and giving me my favorite ice cream bar. He can somehow create a quiet, just-for-the-two-of-us space and do something sweet. Often we have to wait until later, but when he has already lit my pilot light, we have had quickies in the bathroom, running the shower, with the kids on the other side, and he's doing me from behind and we're watching in the mirror." You never know when those opportunities may present themselves to give her your undivided attention, which is so key to relaxing her and getting her in the mood for sex.

4. Make her comfortable. A woman will not relax and let herself be open to getting turned on if she feels self-conscious or bad about her body. Women blossom under attention and positive body comments. Most women, even those with model bodies, question their attractiveness and often have negative

feelings around their body image. I'm assuming since you're with her that you find her attractive and want to be with her. Let her know what you like about her and what you'd like to do to her. She wants and needs to hear that you are attracted to her. A few chosen words from her man have been known to get one woman "so wet, sometimes he does it to me when I am at the office over the phone. He's so bad!" Another woman says she goes absolutely wild when her partner says, "I want my mouth where it was last Friday night."

SECRET FROM LOU'S ARCHIVES
The two biggest robbers of intimacy are being tired and having no time. Early in relationships, you make intimacy a priority, but later, you may let it slide—especially if there are children in the picture. Plainly and simply, you and your partner need to make attending to your intimate relationship a priority.

Have you recently told her about the part of her body you find the biggest turn-on? In a couples seminar a couple who had been married five years with two children shocked each other with their responses. "I love the way the hair curls at the back of her neck and the little dimples above her buttocks." His wife could only say, "You're kidding . . . I hate those," and he said, "I know I love 'em." And then she jerked back and said, "No wonder you like doggy style so much!" In full-throated, blushing laughter he said, "Busted!" For her, his hands were her major turn-on— " 'cause you're big and strong and I love to look at them and remember how they feel on my body." Once she knows how you feel about a part of her beautiful anatomy, remind her, often and regularly.

TIPS TO HELP HER RELAX

➤ Create a space that makes her relax. A woman responds keenly to her environment. Create an oasis for her—whether it's the bedroom, the living room, the outside porch, or the bathroom. Use lighting, scent, or other sensory stimulation to declare that the workday has ended, and now it's time to relax.

➤ Before she walks in the door, draw her a bath. Light candles or incense, help her undress, and sit beside her (on the throne, obviously not using it) so you can share this wind-down time with her. Help bathe her or rub her back with a loofah. Perhaps you want to give her a glass of wine or a cool glass of water. One woman, a children's book illustrator from New Jersey, recalled, "I knew I was marrying my husband the first time he drew a bath for me and bathed me. I wasn't gonna let that one get away. And to this day he loves to wash my hair." The seduction you are offering here is in the fact that you have been thinking of her even before she arrives home. Every woman in the world wants to know in her heart of hearts that he can and will take care of her physically and emotionally, and every woman wants to feel special and appreciated.

➤ Once out of the bath, ask her if she'd like you to give her a pedicure, or towel her off, or offer to rub moisturizing lotion on her. Analogous to the real estate mantra "location, location, location," women want "attention, attention, attention"—in whatever form you can imagine.

Engage Her Five Senses

By enticing her five senses—sight, smell, taste, hearing, and touch—you bring her one step closer to the second element of foreplay, awakening her body. Consider engaging her senses to be the crucial link or bridge that connects her mind to her body. Now that you have romanced her, relaxed her mind, it's time to begin awakening her body. As a CPA from Chicago said, "I want to touch as many of her senses as I can—all of them." Elicit and engage her senses, and she will become putty in your delighted hands.

SIGHT

Humans are essentially visual creatures. As such, sight is one of our most powerful senses because it is the one we rely on most. Men have shared again and again that they like and respond to the way a woman creates a home or an environment that is inviting. So why not capitalize on what you know works and do the same for her? By creating a special, intimate space, you are sure to score points with her.

The visual appeal of your love nest can have a wondrous effect on her, so it's to your advantage if you keep your room, apartment, or house neat and tidy. Please do not ask a lady to sleep in an unmade or already slept-in bed. And clothes strewn about on the floor, bed, or lamp shade are not going to be considered art—believe me. Yuck! She'll think of you as stuck in college. In order to make a woman feel special, invite her into a place that shows you care about yourself.

HELPFUL TIPS
➤ Dim lighting is flattering—to both of you.
➤ If you really want to seduce her, put a discreet bud vase

holding one flower either by the bed or in a place that's visible from the bed. This can be one of your "tonight" signals.

➤ For single men, if you have any photos in your room, make sure they are not of exes—this could be a turnoff.

SMELL

When it comes to eliciting her "scentual" responses, you can use smell, either to engage her or to repel her, so be sure you pay attention here. Smell is one of our most primitive senses, said by some to have the longest recall power. Chances are you have been with a woman who wore a particular scent that to this day you experience a rush of emotion when you smell it. You may have forgotten her face or name, but remember her perfume. Keep in mind, gentlemen, that your own body chemistry may be your greatest asset. You have your own particular scent, which will explain why some people find you irresistible. For some ladies, how you smell is the ultimate pheromone. One woman said, "Oh God, I loved how he smelled. It wasn't his cologne; it was what emanated from his neck. One whiff and I wanted him all over me."

SECRET FROM LOU'S ARCHIVES

A woman's sense of smell is much more sensitive than a man's, and you may not be aware of what scent may be lingering around. A solution is to bathe regularly and use soap in important spots.

On the other hand, men sweat more than women, and as such, they need to be very aware of their hygiene when it involves a lady.

The sweat in the apocrine glands, which are the specialized sweat glands in the armpit and groin, secrete a more viscous and pungent sweat. When this sweat comes into contact with regular body bacteria, the result is body odor. The best way to avoid offending your partner is to shower frequently and use deodorant. Some ladies will be turned on by your natural body scent, but don't confuse this with BO.

SECRET FROM LOU'S ARCHIVES

There are some men that by virtue of their smell alone are irresistible to the women they attract. One woman put it this way: "I loved what my pillows smelled like after he'd slept over. And when he wasn't there I'd have to sleep with one of his old sweaters. It was a major turn-on and soothing."

Since most women respond strongly to scent, a powerful way to engage her is through the practice of aromatherapy. A term coined by a nineteenth-century chemist, R. N. Gattefosse, aromatherapy signifies "the therapeutic use of odiferous substances obtained from flowers, plants and aromatic shrubs, through inhalation and application to the skin." These natural scents come in the form of essential oils for direct application on the skin, as bath salts, or candles. Each scent works on a different area of the body or sensibility.

When used in the sexual arena, these scents can help relax her and heighten her sexual pleasure. According to Valerie Ann Worwood in her book *Scents and Scentuality*, essential oils act *directly* on the brain's olfactory (smell) receptors, which act immediately on the brain's emotional centers, unlike chemical tranquilizers, which act indirectly and must pass through the digestive system or blood before acting on the nervous system.

These scented oils can be used in several ways.

- ➤ Placed on an unscented column candle
- ➤ Dropped into her bath
- ➤ Blended into massage oil
- ➤ Placed in an infuser
- ➤ Carefully placed in drops on a lightbulb

HELPFUL TIPS

- ➤ Check in with her about your aftershave or cologne. Women will be either turned on or turned off by certain scents.
- ➤ Are your linens clean? You may not be aware of your own scent, and though she may like it, it's best always to use fresh sheets.
- ➤ Check your laundry detergent. Some of the name brands carry a very distinctive, not altogether pleasant odor. You may want to consider using a detergent that is scent-free.
- ➤ Check your deodorant. Does it work? Is its scent too over-powering or just right?
- ➤ When using essential oils in any form, make sure never to apply them to her or your genitals.

TASTE

How we taste and what tastes we like are completely individualistic. Yet arousing our taste buds can literally whet the appetite of her and your desire. Have you ever tried feeding her? In bed? Or have her feed you? Grapes can be tons of fun, and if you drop them, it's no big deal. The following foods are widely considered to be some of the best (i.e., most seductive).

Strawberries—whole, dipped in chocolate or dipped in a mixture of sour cream and brown sugar—they're amazing!

Figs—Select fresh, plump figs, whose soft, downy surface may remind her of your testicles. Who knows, you may want to start showing up for dates with some figs instead of a bottle of wine.

Grapes—These delicate little fruits are truly a fun food. Hold one in your mouth and ask her to bite it out.

Plums—They taste best during summer, and these luscious sweet fruits cleanse any palate.

Chocolate—dark, milk, white, in whatever combination you desire. This bit of sweetness can be used as a transitional item, moving you from before sex to sex, as it contains phenylethylamine, the same chemical the brain produces when people fall in love.

Olives—if stuffed with pimiento or an almond, consider having her suck the filling out while you hold the olive in your mouth.

Oysters—in the raw, of course, as they are quite erotic and resemble female genitalia. They also contain a lot of zinc, an important mineral that increases male potency.

Nuts—almonds, Brazil nuts, cashews.

Cheese—some prefer a hard cheese like Jarlsberg, others a smooth-bodied Brie or Camembert.

Beverages—wine (FYI, red wine goes very well with chocolate), champagne, juice, cool water (flat or bubbly).

SECRET FROM LOU'S ARCHIVES

In Chaucerian England, the word "mussel" was a naughty synonym for vulva.

HELPFUL TIPS

➤ Cleanliness of the mouth and body is a given for all involved.

➤ Don't introduce *too* many tastes; otherwise you will overwhelm your taste buds. A sampling of a few items works best—remember, this is an appeteaser.

➤ Remember the basic rule when choosing a beverage: Don't let it overpower or mask the food.

HEARING

Forgive me for repeating myself, but I feel I need to remind you that women can and do get seduced through their ears. Yes, it can be the words you say, but you can also reach her in more subtle ways. Did you know that certain women's clothing stores play low, melodious music in the background, hoping to relax women while they shop? Do you remember the studies that led to Muzak? Both instances point to the powerful, soothing effect of music on the human brain, but especially on women.

SECRET FROM LOU'S ARCHIVES

If your answering machine is in hearing distance of the bedroom, turn the volume off, and if you have a phone by your bed, turn off the ringer. There is no greater mood-shatterer than a ringing phone or the sound of your mother's voice.

In planning a romantic evening or preparing to relax your partner, you may want to consider playing music. Perhaps neither of you wants to listen to music, but rather hear it, gracefully, in the background. Any kind of instrumental music has a calming or soothing effect—even Beethoven's Fifth. Music without words allows the brain to move, wander, and let go of the outside world.

If you're not familiar with instrumental music, try surfing through the classical or jazz section at your local music store. And of course, there is always Barry White, the Master of Seduction, and Marvin Gaye when you already know one another. But be forewarned about listening to Barry or Marvin unless you intend to take action. So for those of you who may want to begin more slowly, you may want to consider these suggestions:

Phillip Aaberg, *Out of the Frame* (New Age)
Enya, *Watermark* (contemporary vocals)
Kenny Rankin, *The Kenny Rankin Album* (contemporary vocals)
Keith Jarrett, *Arbour Zena* (New Age jazz)
John Barry, *Moviola* (contemporary composers)
Windham Hill Retrospective (New Age)
Verve Jazz Round Midnight series, featuring Chet Baker,
    Billie Holiday, and Ben Webster (jazz)

Another way to help relax her through her ears is to try a decorative fountain. Now, I don't mean putting a Trevi-size fountain in the middle of your living room. These decorative fountains are small, and fit easily on top of a stereo speaker, a table, or a bookshelf. Some men and women have remarked that the sound of trickling water in the background helps to decrease their tension as well as increase their sexual appetite.

HELPFUL TIPS
➤ Play music low.
➤ Choose music that has a slow beat or rhythm, until you want
    to switch to the driving beat of "flesh-slapping" music.

- ➤ Ask her if she has any favorite recordings.
- ➤ Suggest selecting music together.

TOUCH

By awakening her four other senses, you are now ready to begin to touch her. As such, the fifth sense is the ultimate bridge from her mind to her body. You may have noticed that women often act like cats when they are being stroked and will curve into your arms and around your body. Any kind of interbody contact will help her relax, which in turn will enable her to become aroused. Not only is touching often the best way to relax a woman, which, again, is absolutely key to both a woman's involvement and her arousal, it is the simplest way for the two of you to connect. "I am that hard-driving successful woman, yet all my husband has to do is touch me in public on the arm or back, as he's walking up from behind. There is something about his touch that is so calming for me. And he has this invisible signal of 'Let's go' or 'Can we be alone?' He gently squeezes my hand. It works wonders at dinner parties."

In the next chapter, we shift focus from her mind to her body. As you begin to travel her body, look for signs of her relaxing: Has her breathing changed? Become deeper? Slower? Gentlemen, keep in mind one simple fact: Once she is relaxed, she's much more likely to unravel in your arms.

—————— • ——————

FOUR

Awakening Her Body's Erogenous Zones

Kiss Her, Touch Her, Tease Her

While romancing and relaxing are what gets her in the mood by putting her mind in a receptive state for sex, this second stage of foreplay is what harnesses and catapults that energy into the stratosphere. Now it's time to take her body and charge it, subtly building the momentum of her sexual stimulation. One woman claims her husband is a magician when it comes to foreplay. "He has this knack for starting foreplay twenty-four hours ahead. He leaves little hints about what he might like to do, what parts of my body he wants to taste, where he wants to do things, and he leaves these on Post-its in my Dayrunner."

In the same way that getting her in the mood requires making her feel special, turning her on physically requires giving her your full attention. If she feels that you are completely engaged in the moment, focused on her, on being with her and pleasing her, she is bound to open like a flower in the midday sun. And isn't her releasing all her inhibitions and letting go what really turns *you* on? In order to let go, however, she needs to feel safe with you. One investment banker from New York remembered this: "The first time my girlfriend really let go and let me reach her sexually was so awesome. I experienced her body and its reactions to me on a completely different level. I had never had that connection with any other woman and that's why we're still together. It was both awesome and something that at the same time stopped my heart."

> **SECRET FROM LOU'S ARCHIVES**
> You don't have to be in the same room or day to begin foreplay.

A woman, a photographer from Washington, D.C., told me this: "My old boyfriend had a way of stopping the world when we made love. He'd get this little smile on his face and lock the front door. There was something about how intense his attention was—that was a major, major turn-on. And everything else on my mind would disappear. It didn't matter that I had to leave for work in thirty minutes. I'd fix my hair in the car."

My point here is twofold. Unless she feels relaxed and comfortable, then nothing you can do will rev her engine. That's why in the previous chapter I provided you with ways to romance and relax her. Now it's time to begin to please her body, and that means kissing her, touching her, and teasing her.

Often women have said they feel their partners only touch them when they want sex. And although this may indeed be your goal, gentlemen, you will get much further if every touch contact doesn't lead to sex. Honest. I am sorry to sound like a broken record on this subject, but it is a common comment I hear from women in the seminars.

As one woman said, "I love him and want to be with him, but why does every touch contact have to be about sex? Sometimes when he just kisses the top of my head or hugs me when he walks by, I feel so loved. It makes me feel *more* open to sex." A man put it this way: "It doesn't take a genius to know that by touching all of her body, you get a sense of how she likes to be touched."

SECRET FROM LOU'S ARCHIVES

The more a man stays in contact with a woman in a nonsexual way, the more receptive she will be to him.

Kiss Her

There is nothing more appealing to most women than the sensuous power of a kiss. Whether that kiss is wet, cool, brief, or lingering, alone it can have the power to bring your lady to her knees. From my observations in women's seminars, I would say that kissing well is the number one indicator of your general prowess as a lover. As one graphic designer from Florida said, "It is the thing that gets my motor running. All the touching in the world cannot take the place of how intensely his kissing turns me on." Another woman remembered an old boyfriend this way: "He loved me and I loved him, but our sexual chemistry never jelled because I hated the way he kissed and he never would listen to the way I wanted to be kissed." Men also remark on the power of kissing. One seminar attendee said, "I find kissing intensely during foreplay very sexy and arousing."

On the other hand, the majority of us have memories of those great kissing episodes when we were younger. Well, let's get serious here. The reason they were such great kissing sessions is that they did what kissing is supposed to do—get everything going. In long-term relationships, it's natural to forget about how wonderful kissing can be. We tend to overlook the skillful kissing that used to really make things happen. If you knew it then, be reminded of that bicycle analogy and know you've still got it.

If you kiss a woman well, and kiss her the way she wants to be kissed, you are halfway to your destination of having her fall into your arms and melt in your mouth. How you kiss her and how she likes to be kissed are important; but more important, I think, is to kiss with feeling and intention. In short, this is where you communicate your love and intimacy. An architect from Coral Gables, Florida, said, "I had always heard about those 'wow,' totally-melt-you kissers and figured, yeah, they're like multiple orgasms. Until I met Stuart. All I can say is this: Kissing him made me leave my body. I can't honestly remember what he even did that sent me through the roof. Well, I can remember one thing: He did this lip-sucking move that to this day makes me wet when I think about it."

SECRET FROM LOU'S ARCHIVES

Some women love to have their tongues gently sucked into your mouth while kissing; others do not. It's always good policy for you to ask her what she likes and what it does for her, and to pay attention to her signals. Note: No human Hoovers please.

The next most important thing to remember is we all have our unique brand of kissing. Sometimes our styles change with our mood; others change with the weather. Regardless, variation is the key. You may want to ask her to "kiss me the way you want me to kiss you." So if she nibbles around the side of your mouth or sucks on your lower lip, definitely ask, "Do you want me to do that to you?"

Here are some helpful tips to keep in mind.

➤ A woman with a pouty, full lower lip probably likes having it sucked slowly and sweetly into your mouth.

➤ Try running the curved tip of your tongue along the inside of her upper lip. The underside of your tongue will be against her teeth, with your taste-bud side against the inner part of her upper lip. Again, not all women like this, so ask her.

➤ Have both of you suck on one another's tongue. "He had a way of sucking on my tongue. He'd do it slowly, then kiss me, then again, then suck me right in, then just the tip . . ."

➤ Please don't push your entire tongue into a woman's mouth—unless you know she wants you to. Chances are your tongue is bigger than hers. One woman said it felt like "he was shoving his tongue down my throat."

➤ Be aware of how loose your lips are. If they are too loose, they will feel sloppy to her.

➤ Avoid the Woody Woodpecker kissing technique, which entails a pointy-tongued devil who darts his stiff tongue in and out in an awkward semblance of French kissing.

➤ Best to adopt the tortoise strategy, not that of the hare. Relative to speed, slow and steady kissing will win the race.

SECRET FROM LOU'S ARCHIVES

A brochure published in 1936 stated that kissing can lead to pregnancy—indirectly, as we know, but effectively nonetheless.

KISSES

The French Kiss. This kiss, also known as soul kissing, takes its name from the British and American soldiers during World War II who attributed anything sexually liberated to the French. This is by far the most widely known kind of kiss. A good French kiss can last for hours. Here, rhythm is everything. You need to alternate your rhythm, suck on her tongue, and move your tongue around. Be careful to avoid sucking on her tongue too hard or making your tongue too pointy (known as the Woody Woodpecker).

The Swoon. I've heard from my sources (the seminars) that one of the most seductive ways to kiss a woman is for the man, while he is standing in front of her, to cradle her head and neck with his hands so her head relaxes into his hands.

The Up-Against-the-Wall Kiss. Sometimes this is one of the hottest types of kisses because it is the most urgent and ardent. You can lean your body against hers with your arms on the wall on either side of her, or she can lean into you.

The Stairs. This position is for those times when you want to be eye-to-eye, if there is a height difference. She may also respond to this position if she wants to see how it feels to tower over you. One man said that "on our first date when we were kissing good night my girlfriend looked up at me and said, 'I want to try something.' Holding my shoulders, she walked to the stairs and stood so we were at eye level and said, 'Good. I just wanted to level the playing field.' She then proceeded to kiss me. Her being in charge really turned her on."

The Kiss-Anytime Card. Use this card, similar to a Get out of Jail Free card from Monopoly, to spice up your love life. Since it never expires, you can leave it somewhere, send it, or deliver it personally. The card can have the kind of kiss you really want to deliver.

A Not-on-the-Mouth Kiss. Use your lips to their best advantage by kissing all over her entire body. As you know, her body is an enchanted forest you want to get lost in, with plenty of unexplored territory. You may want to try the insides of her arms, upper shoulders, buttocks, backs of her knees, armpits, and everywhere else.

The Picasso. Many women also like a form of genital kissing. As one gentleman from my seminar said, "I love to kiss a woman 'down there,' her nipples, or anywhere, and then go back to her mouth." For some women, your tasting her and being that open about it is a special act of acceptance—one of the most powerful aphrodisiacs and akin to a lady tasting and/or swallowing you.

> **SECRET FROM LOU'S ARCHIVES**
> Kissing is the number one way to get your lady's motor running.

The Hand Kiss. One of the more gracious forms of courtly behavior. When she extends her hand as if to have you shake it, grasp it lightly, just as you would if you were going to shake it. Then turn it clockwise and kiss the back of her hand in the middle, making sure your lips are dry. Hold the kiss for two seconds, then release her hand. One woman recounted this story: "On our second date, we had just ordered the wine. When the sommelier had left, my boyfriend turned to me and said, 'I have wanted to do this all night.' Then, ever so gently, he picked up my left hand and, raising it to his lips, softly and very slowly kissed the back of my hand. Oh migod, he couldn't have done anything more seductive and understated."

Touch Her

Here is where we return to the fifth sense. When you are touching all areas of her body, overlook no surface. One man has said after giving his partner a massage, "I know I've done a good job when she's almost asleep or she gets mad when I finish."

Of course, every woman is different and you may want to adhere to the cardinal rule of "ask first." It's also just as important for you to enjoy her whole body. As one woman warned, "I felt like I was a machine with operating parts. He'd touch A then B then C and I was supposed to be ready for sex. My God—enough already. I'm not on remote control." That said, the key to amazing foreplay is in your willingness to travel her body, caressing it while at the same time staying away from the so-called action spots (i.e., her genitals).

You may also want to keep in mind that the majority of us will touch someone the way we like to be touched. But very often there is a difference between the pressure a man likes and what a woman likes. Men tend to prefer deeper, stronger pressure, while women respond more to gentler, softer pressure. Why? Because as a function of testosterone, the male hormone, a man's skin is thicker and denser.

As a result, the touch that works for you may be too firm for her and may make her feel uncomfortable or actually hurt her.

Gentlemen, I know you may not be comfortable with asking or receiving directions, so I have provided you with a topographical guide, so to speak, of a woman's body. What I have heard again and again from men in my seminars is that you truly respond to maps and guides, liking to peruse them at your leisure, in order to familiarize yourselves with various routes or the logistics of a trip. I am going to be systematic here and start at the top of her body and move down, giving you hints and pointers about how to enliven each particular area.

HEAD

The majority of women like to have their head massaged and their hair touched, played with, and enjoyed. Remember the feeling of a good scalp massage? You need to employ that same kind of motion to your lover's head. You may want to do this on a night that you are not going out and she doesn't mind having her hair mussed up.

You may also want to try running your fingertips or a hairbrush through her hair gently and steadily. If you have a daughter or a sister whose hair you have brushed, you may be at an advantage in this area. Although the stroke can be a straight, downward motion, you can give yourself some varying moves by doing a J-shaped stroke, which is a long stroke through her hair with a little up tail at the end. Remember to brush her entire head, not just the back. You might also ask her to brush yours to show you how she likes her own hair brushed. This way, you can study how she varies the stroke, its location, and its strength.

TIPS
- Gently play with her hair at the base of her neck, lift it, and kiss underneath.
- Hold her against you and let her feel your warm breath on her scalp; this will be subtle but deeply felt.
- If your arm is around her shoulders, play with her hair as you walk.

SECRET FROM LOU'S ARCHIVE
According to a hairstylist who could have been the model for Warren Beatty's character in *Shampoo,* the more hair on the nape of a woman's neck, the more abundant her pubic hair—some men love lots of pubic hair, and some men just don't. It's all individualistic.

FACE
Face touching is a very gentle, intimate gesture, and the key to making it as sensual as possible is the intensity of eye-to-eye contact. But be aware of whether or not she is wearing makeup. If she is, ask her to remove it, then use the back of your hand or finger to trace lightly

the side of her jawline, down her cheekbone, and then down her neck. Believe me, women remember how you touch them.

TIPS

➤ Use the tips of your fingers to outline her lips. Close both your eyes and do the same to each other.

➤ Ask her to suck on your finger once it is close to her mouth. An interested lady will show you on your finger what else her tongue can do, and you can use this as a prelude to using your tongue elsewhere.

➤ Play a game in which each of you, eyes closed, kisses the other *just* on the side of the mouth. If your nose touches, you lose.

EARS

Remember how we spoke of being able to tell how your lover likes being touched by how she touches you? Well, the way in which a woman responds to touching of her ear is a perfect example of how men and women differ. As one male seminar attendee said, "A woman who puts her tongue in my ear is a straight-line boner for me." This makes sense, as men's ears are an androgenic receptor site; in other words, those cells receive signals from the male hormones, which is the reason men have hair in their ears.

For the majority of women, however, a tongue in the ear is like having their head in a washing machine. (There are, however, women who love this sensation, but they are definitely in the minority.) The action I am referring to here is glomming onto her ear with suction and pushing your tongue into the ear. It's best to use your full wet mouth on other parts of her body, not at this tender conical opening. If you can't resist her ear, best to try tracing along the outside rim and behind the back of her earlobe with your tongue or sucking on her earlobes. Be sure to use a full open mouth for a less direct, warm breath.

TIPS

➤ Breathe lightly. She wants to know you are there, but you don't want to risk sounding like a hurricane.

➤ Be careful not to blow too forcefully into her ear; if too harsh, this move, while tempting in a romantic kind of way, will not arouse her.

➤ Lick, then lightly blow. This technique causes the opposing sensations of heat/moisture and then cooling. You may also want to try this on her nipples, side of her neck, or the curve of her back.

NECK AND SHOULDERS

This erogenous zone is invariably a doozy for women. Touching her neck and shoulders can create goose bumps and shivers all over her body if done in the right way. It's best to use a circular, wavy motion rather than a straight up-and-down motion. Your tongue, lips, fingers, and chin will work well for you here. She is more than likely going to respond like a cat and nuzzle into you. Her skin here is very sensitive and thin, so you don't need to use a lot of pressure. As one woman said, "When he starts down my neck, I can feel my crotch heat up. I can't believe such a small area can cause my whole body to react. I shiver all over."

The adage that variety is the spice of life is very true here. Don't always use the same motion. Make your fingers and hands continue down to her shoulders. Balance your touch on both sides—don't overlook what massage therapists have known for years!

TIPS
- The sides of a woman's neck from the base of her earlobes to the top of her neck are one of the more sensitive areas on her body.
- Start softly with fingertips, mix in lips and tongue, and be sure to touch both sides.
- Lift up her hair and kiss down the back of her neck, and continue across her shoulders. This is a perfect move when she's wearing anything strapless.

SECRET FROM LOU'S ARCHIVES

Ladies have asked that you please don't go directly to action spots. Instead, delay arrival. They prefer a slow buildup. Paying attention to the minor areas first is critical.

BELLY BUTTON

Some women love to have a tongue, finger, or nose in their belly button. For others this is decidedly not the case. "I love it when he plays with my belly button ring, because his mouth is hot. He says he likes that side of me—I'm an executive by day and a club girl by night." Another woman, a mother of three, said, "No way. Poking anything in it makes me want to pee."

TIPS
- All points from the top of the pubic hair to the point between the breasts can be massaged in a gentle, circular (clockwise) motion with fingers or thumbs.

➤ Consider her belly button the perfect repository for champagne or other beverages. As it is just north of a highly enervated area, any attention to her navel will spread there.

BACK

The area across her back right above the curve of her buttocks, which is called the sacral curve, is often a very sensitive pressure zone. By gently applying pressure with your entire hand, you may excite her in a way mysterious to you both. Stroking the whole of her back or lightly tracing the area with your fingers is another inventive move. As one lady said, "This is why you have hot breath and why we women wear backless gowns."

TIPS

➤ Some women may be self-conscious of your attention to this area because of its proximity to her derriere, so be considerate and aware. Either tell her how much you enjoy touching this area, or, if she's too sensitive, concentrate on the front of her body.

➤ Moving from her back down to her buttocks brings sensation from her groin into her genital area.

➤ One way to build lubrication is to focus on the small dimples on her back. Tell her what you're going to do and then put your tongue there.

BUTTOCKS

Dare we overlook one of men's more admired areas of a woman's body? As I mentioned above, many women are sensitive or uncomfortable about not only exposing but having their derrieres be the center of attention. It's up to you to show and tell her that you love her buttocks. One woman from a seminar said, "When my boyfriend told me that part of me is the one part he loves to watch, touch, and taste, I was astounded. Now that I'm more comfortable, we read the Sunday paper and he rests his head in the curve of my back with his cheek on the curve of my butt."

TIPS

➤ If you position your lady on all fours, you can lean your chest against her buttocks and caress her breasts at the same time.

➤ If she enjoys anal play, you can begin to heighten her sensation by gently spreading her cheeks; this will stimulate her anus, reminding her of things to come.

LIMBS

Think of all the room you have here! Legs, arms, wrists, hands! As with any touching, be sure to touch both sides of her, as balancing sensation is important. When it comes to touching her limbs, you can use more pressure because the skin is thicker. Recently on a plane, I watched a couple as the woman leaned into him, half asleep. Her partner was gently circling her hand and wrist with his fingertips, and judging from the serene smile on her face, she was in bliss. It was sweet to watch him watching her. He was making her feel so good.

TIPS

➤ Touching her limbs is a great way to enliven her nerve endings, creating radiating pleasure in the outer reaches of her body.

➤ The other benefit to touching limbs is they are external—you can have as much fun as you want in public! Limbs are also a great place to do the Swirl (see later in this chapter).

FEET

In this area of the body, I have borrowed from the Chinese, who have used the feet as the entryway to the rest of the body. When rubbing or massaging a woman's feet, there are a couple of important things to remember. You both need to be in a comfortable position in which you can access both feet easily. Try sitting between her legs on the floor in front of her, or with her leg draped over yours as you face her toes. Use a body lotion to give you greater ease of stroking motion and drape a towel over your knee so no lotion lands where it shouldn't.

The main aim in a foot massage is to release the tension of the tiny muscles and ligaments holding the little bones in place. Your thumbs will be your best digits for foot massages. It's best to use small circular strokes from the heel up to the toes with both thumbs, the way a masseur would move up your spine. Don't use a two-handed squeeze from the instep up to the toes. Any compacting, squishing motion pushes all the little bones in the foot together, and that hurts. If she is close to getting her period, the outer side below her ankle may be very tender. Be gentle. Release toe pressure by gently pulling each toe in an upward motion. Start with your thumbs together at the center of the bottom of the foot and, using an outward stroking motion with both thumbs, firmly stroke across the ball of the foot. Use that same stroke all the way down the foot, top and bottom. Next use the heel of your hand on her heel in a circular motion and then switch to your thumb or your index and middle fingers, bent like little knees, for more intense pressure. And of course there is the sucking on her toes and/or any other oral play.

According to Valerie Ann Worwood, author of *Scents and Scentuality*, the foot contains a number of erotic trigger points, which, when pressed, will create sensation in a woman's genitals.

➤ Massage the big toes with thumb and fingers.

➤ Massage three inches along either side of the bone running from the back of the heel up toward the calf of the leg.

➤ Use a circular massage technique to connect the three points that run in a line from the end of the heel to the sole of the foot to the crease by the middle toe. You can also connect the fourth point on the sole, just inside the bridge.

Massaging these points, based loosely on reflexology (see foot diagram), will

1. Increase relief.
2. Reduce anxiety.
3. Clear the mind.

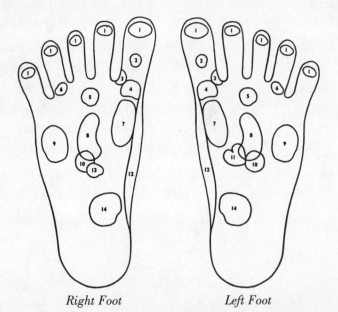

Right Foot   *Left Foot*

Reflexology Chart

4. Reduce neck tension.
5. Reduce eye stress.
6. Improve mood.
7. Reduce stress.
8. Regulate breathing.
9. Reduce tension.
10. Reduce nervousness.
11. Increase circulation.
12. Loosen stomach muscles.
13. Reduce anxiety.
14. Reduce nervousness.

BREASTS

Some women love to be touched here and others don't. One woman in my seminar really doesn't like having her breasts massaged. "I'd rather take a cold bath," she says. For her, it's just not pleasurable. But other women love it! They love to have their breasts cradled, sucked, and played with. One male surgeon who attended a seminar said the woman he dated wanted her nipples bitten, and while doing her bidding, he thought he was going to bite them off. Someone's *ouch* may be another's *mmmmm*.

It is best to start from underneath and gently move toward the nipples. Like just about everything else, women need you to build toward the center of interest, and that includes nipples. The straight-to-the-nipples approach doesn't allow a woman time to relax into the sensation. And FYI, the majority of ladies *do not* enjoy intense pinching of their nipples. It is "like rubbing a cat the wrong way—and you are likely to get the same result—pissing her off." Also, the grab and squeeze technique is best left in the greengrocer's. Breasts may be shaped like oranges, but they rarely appreciate the squeeze test.

Again, it's up to you to experiment and discover how she likes to be touched. You may want to ask her to guide your hands by putting hers over the top of yours and showing you how she wants you to do things. You may also consider watching her masturbate, assuming

---

SECRET FROM LOU'S ARCHIVES

A physician told me that women who come in for mammograms regularly say it was their boyfriends or husbands who found the lump or odd-feeling tissue. Here is a very good opportunity to help women's health by paying close attention to a woman's breasts. It's best, however, to choose the same time of the month to do the exam, as any changes caused by the monthly hormonal cycle will be the same.

---

she is comfortable with that. Does she flick her own nipple with a finger or hold the entire breast? Does she pull them up toward her face or cup them together?

If she enjoys intense nipple pressure once she is stimulated, you might try using nipple clips with adjustable tension. If none are available, bobby pins and clothespins are excellent substitutes.

THE SWIRL AND SENSUAL MASSAGE

Now that you have been introduced to the body's erogenous zones, here are two ways to put all that information together. The first method is called the Swirl, which is a light touch enveloping her entire body. The second method is what I call the Sensual Massage, which is the same movement with more pressure and using both your hands at the same time.

THE SWIRL

A woman's skin is her largest sexual organ—despite what you may have heard to the contrary. As a result, anywhere that she has skin can become an erogenous zone, depending on how you touch, caress, and pamper her. Think of it this way: If you're in a boardroom sitting next to a woman you find attractive, and your elbows happen to touch, chances are you remember it, right? In my seminars, I suggest that men first see how this move feels on themselves. So, using the front of your thigh as the practice field (you can do this with or without vêtements), scratch in a straight line from your knee to the groin. Do the stroke first with nails, and then with just your fingertips, to see the difference. Then do it again, varying the pressure. Immediately cover the same field using a wavy, undulating stroke. See the difference? The reason it feels so different is that the little nerves "know" they are getting sensation with the straight line, whereas with the wavy stroke the little nerves are anticipating and hoping they're next. As many men and women have noted, you can do this anywhere on the body with just a simple hand motion.

You can also use the Swirl as a transitional move to the action spots. Let your fingers make her moan for you. Another important feature of the Swirl is that it can be done in many public places without embarrassing her or you by getting you overly excited.

SENSUAL MASSAGE

There is an entire world of sensual massage and many books devoted strictly to the subject. I'm going to provide you with some of the highlights. These techniques do not require much preparation or learning, and they all rely on one simple premise: that you get into it.

Using both hands, gently but steadily apply pressure to the different parts of her body. I think it's always best to start at the top (her head) and work down (to her feet). Don't include her breasts or her groin area—the so-called action spots. These are too sensitive and may create an uncomfortable amount of sexual tension, thereby undermining the point of the massage.

Depending on how sensitive she is, vary and gauge the degree of pressure. Here are some important tips:

- ➤ Always balance what you do on one side by repeating the move on the other side.
- ➤ Use lotion or massage oil so that your hands move easily over her skin. Reapply as often as needed.
- ➤ Pour the lotion or oil into your hands and rub them together. This is a way to avoid touching her with cold hands.
- ➤ Use a towel or sheet to cover the parts of her body that you are not touching, and make sure the room is warm.
- ➤ Choose soothing music.

Tease Her

Kiss her, touch her, and now you're ready to push her over the edge. When teasing is subtle, with a precise purpose and direction (i.e., to make her swoon), then, gentlemen, it is totally legal. So for those of you who are wanting to perfect the art of the tease, I have gathered some information taken from the hundreds of women with whom I have spoken in the course of writing first the ladies' book and now this one. After all, isn't our goal here to give her and you absolute pleasure?! The power of teasing is in the mysterious interplay of her mind and body. Here are some reported teasing delights.

1. Compose a fantasy scenario together. You write one line/paragraph and she writes the next one.

2. Share one of your fantasies in which she is featured. If you're afraid you may shock her with your fantasy's frankness, you might edit it lightly, while you feel her out and see how she reacts.

3. Call her on the phone from work and tell her what you want to do to her that night.

4. Leave her a voice mail describing what you want to do to her, or read her a piece of erotica and leave it on voice mail.

5. Use the lovely ritual of dining to build up the tension between you. One woman shared her and her husband's style of public foreplay: "It started because I had recently had surgery on my wrist. We went out for dinner and I was rather helpless, something I never am. My husband all of a sudden got 'that' look in his eyes over the menu and said, 'Let me order for you and feed you.' So when the waiter returned, my husband concocted a story about my situation, ordered, and then scooted up beside me on the U-shaped banquette. The next two hours were so sensual and so sexual. It was such a turn-on having him pay that much attention to me, and it was so sweet when he cut up my food and made it into little-girl size." If you're uncomfortable with a too-public display, just eat and drink slowly, savoring each bite or sip. Believe me: If you pay attention, so will she.

6. Send her a postcard and write down what part of her body most excites you.

Checklist for Fantastic Foreplay

➤ Orgasm is not the only road to satisfaction; how you make one another feel is.

➤ Use lubricant and keep it nearby—on the bedside table or other appropriate place.

➤ Make sure your breath and mouth are clean. I know that's obvious but just to be sure.

➤ Slowly, slowly, slowly.

➤ Involve her entire body. Put your mouth and hands everywhere and use the Swirl.

➤ Using that most powerful of your sex organs, your brain, consider approaching her body as if it or some part of it is new for you. Anyone can say, "Yeah, been there done that," and what shows up is a "been there done that" attitude. If on the other hand you have a fresh new attitude, she will be able to tell. Add that to the comfort of already knowing one another and you have a whole new world to play in. Mentally treat her as new.

➤ Check ideas on yourself first.

➤ Check in with her regularly about pressure and speed, as her preferences can change throughout a given session.

➤ Check stubble. Men with beards can make their beards softer and more user-friendly with hair conditioner.

➤ If one of you is eating spicy or heavily seasoned food prior to being intimate, share a taste with the other. This tip was from an elegant European woman who said in her thick Hungarian accent, "You both need to so your chemistries will blend better." So be sure to share that Caesar salad.

Foreplay, Some Final Words

Fabulous foreplay is all about enticing and exciting both her mind and her body. I think it's about time, though, that we come up with another term for foreplay. I think this term implies that foreplay isn't enough in and of itself. To the contrary, for women, the kissing, touching, and teasing are necessary and often very satisfying parts of lovemaking. As you will see in the next two chapters on manual and oral sex, women often have trouble letting go if they're not already warmed up. As one woman, a magazine writer from Philadelphia, said, "When we have the time during lovemaking to really play, it is sex on a different plane."

———— • ————

FIVE

Let Your Hands Delight Her

Her Action Spots

I call this chapter and the next the finesse chapters—the place where the men who want to be expert lovers learn to stand out from the crowd. Although we've discussed the power of touching her erogenous zones in arousing her, we haven't yet focused on her action spots. Referring to some of these techniques, one woman asked, "Couldn't you please tell me where you are having the men's seminar so I can wait outside the door and drop my hanky?" It's not the picking up of the hanky that she was after, though that would have been a nice opener. What this woman was really looking for was a man who knew his stuff and was confident enough to know there is always more to know.

There's no doubt about it: Most women love to be touched genitally. In the same way that you enjoy being stroked, coddled, and sometimes even squeezed, women become gloriously aroused when your fingers and hands pay attention to them.

Your typical woman enjoys, and sometimes relies on, genital

touching to get her wet, and ready for penetration or orgasm. You will learn techniques and approaches that will make a lady more comfortable, especially in asking her what she wants when she's not sure what that is. We women are thankful you ask what we like, but sometimes, gentlemen, *we* don't even know. A seminar attendee from San Diego, who is now in her mid-thirties, said that it was her husband, whom she'd met when she was just out of college, who taught her about her own body. Growing up in a conservative Catholic family where it was not okay to talk about sex, never mind learn about her own body, she didn't even know what felt pleasurable until her husband touched her. The key here is that women need your participation and may welcome it more than you ever expected.

SECRET FROM LOU'S ARCHIVES

According to *Science* magazine, a physical skill takes six hours to sink in. After learning a physical skill, such as a variation on your golf stroke or a variation of your cunnilingus stroke, it takes six hours for the info to be stored in permanent memory. But interrupt the storage process by learning another new skill and that first lesson could be erased.

To some women, your hand or mouth on her genitals is more intimate than sexual intercourse. They are allowing you access to the most intimate and private part of themselves and they are doing so in a receiving position, which makes them feel vulnerable. Many women have been culturally programmed to be the giver, not the receiver. Men have told me that it is very important for them to realize that this most intimate of acts can take women some getting used to.

However, if a woman isn't comfortable being touched genitally, she should be respected for her likes and dislikes.

In terms of what works best physically, there is truly a buffet of moves and ideas to consider when touching a woman's genitals. Some women prefer that you start out with a soft, barely-touching tapping on the clitoris. Other women don't want you to go near the "lovebud" until she is much more stimulated. On the other end of the continuum are the women who love very firm, direct, and fast touching directly on the clitoris and all around the area. Other ladies prefer a very specific repetitive, subtle touch. Again, the best guide for you is her. If you already know the oral moves that work for her, try mimicking them as best you can with moistened fingers. Your fingers will create a different sensation, yet you will still have the memory to draw on. A musician from Seattle said, "Learning what a woman likes is like learning to play a completely new instrument. You have working knowledge of the chords for x, but this is y, and it takes practice, practice, practice to feel comfortable and get to where you know what you're doing."

SECRET FROM LOU'S ARCHIVES
Although watching a woman masturbate will definitely give you ideas, you will still not be touching her as she touches herself. Instead, best directions will come from her guiding your hand.

Getting Started

The absolute key to perfecting your ability to arouse her to heights of pleasure with your hands and fingers is knowing how and where to touch her. Without a doubt, if you don't know where you're going, you won't know what to do once you've arrived. With that in mind, I have provided you with another guide so that you will not feel like you're lost in the wilderness. I've also offered some helpful tips on lubrication. These hints apply not only to manual stimulation but also to oral and anal sex as well as intercourse.

Before letting your fingers do the talking, please wash your hands. There are two main reasons. First, the mucosal tissue of a woman's genital area is extremely delicate, and second, the natural salt in the sweat of your fingers can make that area feel like it's burning. And trust me, if that happens, she's not feeling good. The solution is to wash your hands and get all soap off (a liquid antibacterial soap like Purrel will sting like soap). Lick your fingers if there is no water around or use a diaper wipe.

Watch your nails. As one woman said, "Man, when he hits me with his nail, all I can think of is when he's going to hit me again. There is no way I can relax after that." This is a clear signal that at no time will a manicure be more appreciated. A manicure is, without a doubt, the sign of a well-groomed, confident man. Trust me, ladies do look at your hands, not just for the urban legend reasons associated with genital dimension but also to imagine what your hands would feel like on their bodies. If they see jagged, bit-off nails, your appeal factor may drop significantly. And no woman wants a man with dirty fingernails to touch her!

Use lotion if you have or tend to have rough hands. Remember, a lady's skin is not as thick as yours. Calluses may scratch her and will feel rough against her skin. One woman told me, "My husband works with his hands and he used to scratch my skin when he touched me. Now he knows that a foot massage is the best thing to relax me and get me in the mood, so when I walk in the room with the lotion, he knows he's likely to 'get some.' I get my foot massage, he softens his big ol' rough hands, and things just happen from there. Brilliant, huh?"

Her Genitalia

I am presuming you're familiar with the nuts and bolts of this region, but I thought you might welcome some extra information so you *really* understand what you're touching, where women want you to touch them, and in some cases, how you might want to touch them for her maximum benefit and your maximum results. Let me be frank here. It is not unusual for men to be found rooting around in the dark in this area. A woman's body is a bit mysterious—ofttimes for us, as much for you. Most noticeable of the physical differences between men and women is the fact that male genitals are in full view, up front and center, while some of the most important parts of a woman's genitalia can be seen only if the woman spreads her legs. And this applies only to the external genitalia. She also has internal genitalia.

Despite the differences, a woman's genitalia in many ways corresponds to your own. In fact, up until six to eight weeks there is no difference between the XX (female) embryo and XY (male) embryo. We all start out female in utero. It is during the embryonic stage, at about eight weeks, that the production of the male hormone testosterone starts. The addition of testosterone turns the potential labia into a scrotum and the potential clitoris into the head of a penis.

VULVA

The entire area of the external female genital anatomy is called the vulva. The mons pubis is an area of fatty tissue that forms a soft mound over the pubic bone. The mons is covered by skin and pubic hair. The labia majora (often called the outer lips) extend down from the mons to below the vaginal opening. These consist of a fold of skin on each side filled with fatty tissue, sweat and oil glands, and nerve endings. The two outer lips usually meet and cover the urinary and vaginal opening when the woman is not aroused or has her legs together. The labia minora (the inner lips) are inside the outer lips and extend from just above the clitoris to below the vaginal opening. These two folds of skin are thinner and do not have pubic hair or fatty tissue, but they have more nerve endings than the outer lips. Even though they are called "inner," it is not unusual for them to protrude beyond the outer lips.

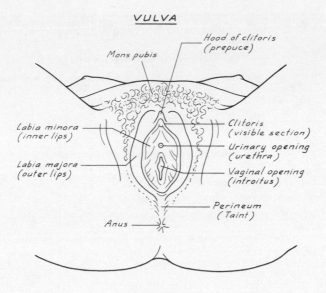

VULVA

Mons pubis

Hood of clitoris
(prepuce)

Labia minora
(inner lips)

Clitoris
(visible section)

Urinary opening
(urethra)

Labia majora
(outer lips)

Vaginal opening
(introitus)

Perineum
(Taint)

Anus

The Vulva

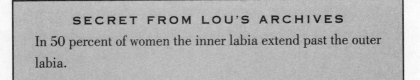

The color of the genitalia varies among women (pink, red, purple, and black are all normal) and may change during arousal. As men's genitalia differ in size, shape, and color, so do the labia minora and majora vary in size, shape, and degree of sensitivity. The head (or glans) of the clitoris is just below where the inner lips meet at the top and is covered with a small fold of skin, the prepuce (equivalent to the foreskin/prepuce in an uncircumcised man). It is a small, sensitive organ at the upper end of the vulva, made up of tissue, blood vessels, and nerves. Hooded by skin, it looks like a tiny dot to the naked eye, but, in fact, most of the clitoris is internal,

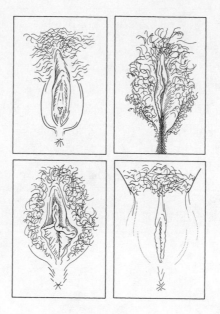

Different Female Genitalia

not external. According to research done by Dr. Helen O'Connell, Urological Surgeon at the Royal Melbourne Hospital in Australia, "the external tip of the clitoris or glans connects on the inside to a pyramid shaped mass of erectile tissue, far larger than previously described. The 'body' of the clitoris, which connects to the glans, is about as big as the first joint of your thumb. It has two arms (or legs) up to nine centimeters long that flare backwards into the body, lying just a few millimeters from the ends of the muscles that run up the inside of the thigh. Also extending from the body of the clitoris, and

---

SECRET FROM LOU'S ARCHIVES

Like an iceberg, most of the clitoris is hidden inside the body.

---

filling the space between the arms, are two bulbs, one on each side of the vaginal cavity."

During sexual stimulation, the pelvic region fills with blood, and the clitoral "tip" swells and becomes firm. This is why after you have stimulated the area, a woman's clitoris is harder to find and doesn't seem as prominent. Like the penis, it has engorged with blood, become erect, and lifted under the prepuce. Since the "clitoral legs" run (see figure 5.3) underneath the labia, any stimulation to the urethral, vaginal, or anal areas will indirectly stimulate the clitoral body as well. This forking of the clitoral legs down and under either side of

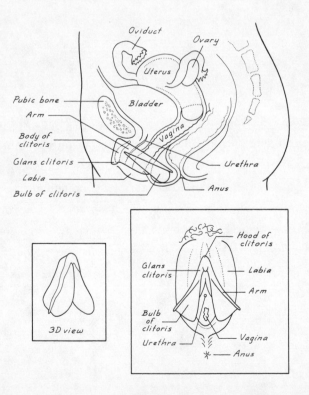

The Clitoris

the labia explains why for some women the most pleasurable use of a vibrator isn't directly on the clitoral bud. They say it is too intense. Rather, holding it against the side of the labia, pressing on the fatty tissue of the outer labia, reaches a broader field of the clitoris with less intense vibration.

SECRET FROM LOU'S ARCHIVES

The clitoris takes its name from the Greek *kleitoris*, which means "little hill."

Just below the clitoral tip is the very small urinary opening, the urethra, and below that is the entrance to the vagina. When you see how close these two openings are, it is easier to understand why so many women experience urinary tract infection after having sex. The infection is a result of new and different bacteria being introduced into the urethra due to the rubbing and thrusting action of intercourse. Hence the term "honeymooner's disease" for this condition, cystitis.

SECRET FROM LOU'S ARCHIVES

The Latin *mons veneris* means "mound of Venus," for the Roman goddess of love.

Below the vaginal opening and where the labia meet is a small area of smooth, usually hairless skin called the perineum. And below that is the anus. This entire perineal area can be very sensitive to stimulation (as it often is in men). Sometimes it's called the taint— "'tain't one, 'tain't the other." One seminar attendee called it the Veranda, and suggests sucking on it or massaging it with your fingers. Some women love the sensation!

VAGINA

Let me start this way: You cannot see the vagina, as it is on the inside of the woman's body. This can be confusing. As I've just described, the vulva and outer labia are visible with the naked eye, but the vagina is not. It's also true that the vagina changes in size and shape, according to the stage of a woman's arousal. It was once described for me this way: "Imagine you are slipping the best part of you into a warm, wet, very soft leather glove. It's the combination of the heat, the pressure, and the moisture that makes it so amazing."

The vagina begins in a constricted state, and when a woman is stimulated mentally, visually, or physically, she will start lubricating within thirty seconds. Just because she is lubricated, however, does not mean that she is "ready" for pentration—whether with your fingers or your penis. Instead, the biggest indicator that a woman is relaxed is her breathing. The deeper it becomes, the more relaxed she is.

SECRET FROM LOU'S ARCHIVES

The vagina lubricates and relaxes, allowing for deeper penetration and deposit of the sperm near the cervix. Mother Nature knew what she was doing in the design category. The penis and vagina make an amazingly great fit! Not that I had to tell you.

In an unaroused state, the vagina is a tube about three to four inches long, which is why an average, five-inch erect penis feels like enough for most women. The vagina is made of muscle and ridged on the inner surface with rugae, or little ridges, and is covered on the inside walls with a mucosal surface—similar to the lining of the mouth. This is the surface that produces the vaginal lubrication. Unless a woman is sexually aroused, the vaginal walls touch each other. Any woman who has inserted a tampon knows this—it feels much tighter than when she is aroused and a penis is inside of her. When a woman becomes aroused, the walls of the vagina produce a slippery liquid and the vaginal walls balloon open so that a penis will fit inside, and, of course, they can be stretched even more during birth.

The degree of a woman's tightness is related to the tightness of the pubococcygeal (PC) muscles at the opening of her vaginal barrel. (The rest of the vaginal barrel expands to accommodate the penis.) The appearance and texture of vaginal secretions vary throughout each monthly reproductive cycle as conditions inside the vagina respond to changes in hormonal levels. This will account for changes in discharge and the woman's natural lubrication. Menopausal and postmenopausal women also have variances in their lubrication.

Other factors also affect a woman's ability to self-lubricate, including alcohol and medications, which can dehydrate the body. In general, a woman's vagina is one of the most self-maintaining and self-cleansing areas of the body. Semen naturally flows out of it, and with regular bathing and cleansing of the labial areas it requires little else. Unless directed otherwise by a physician, there is no need to douche. Besides being unnecessary, douching can be harmful and is the number one cause of bladder and vaginal infections in the United States. As an ob-gyn said, "Women who douche pay my mortgage."

THE G-SPOT

The G-spot was first recognized by the gynecologist Ernst Grafenberg. But it was Dr. John D. Perry and Dr. Beverly Whipple who named it the G-spot after Dr. Grafenberg. The G-spot is yet another nonvisible part of a woman's anatomy. It is located in the tissue above the vaginal wall surrounding the urethra, the tummy side. An area of soft, often ridgy tissue, the G-spot is about the size of a dime when unstimulated and when stimulated swells to the size of a quarter.

SECRET FROM LOU'S ARCHIVES

One man described the G-spot this way: "Sometimes it has felt like a bean, sometimes like a pea. It starts off smooth and gets 'textury.'"

Some women are capable of orgasming with direct stimulation of this area, which may result in a woman's ejaculating, which I go into further in Chapter Eight when I describe female orgasms. The source of the female ejaculation is the paraurethral glands, which are located on either side of the urethra, which is why some people think that the fluid is urine. The paraurethral glands act like a salivary gland, squirting or expressing fluid when stimulated. All women have this urethral sponge or G-spot, but not all respond in the same way to its stimulation. Some women find their G-spot feels no different from other parts of the vaginal barrel; for others, stimulating this dime-size area can send them through the rafters. Yet, again, the difficulty can be in locating it. I know a sex therapist who even had difficulty locating her own G-spot, despite being very comfortable with her body and aware of all her parts. She had to have her partner show her where it was. Truly, in some cases, it's like trying to find the Holy Grail, but if you are patient and sensitive, between the two of you, I trust you will be able to find her G-spot.

Lubrication

Lubrication is one of mankind's greatest inventions, and you should use it to your heart's content. As one mortgage broker from Cleveland said, "I had no idea there was so much fun in one of those little bottles." Sometimes both men and women tend to shy away from using a lubricant, as if the very existence of this slippery, slidy, marvelous stuff were some kind of reflection on their lack of sexual prowess. After his girlfriend attended one of my seminars, a man called and asked me why his partner would be needing "that stuff." I knew that he was really asking, "What am I not doing to get her turned on enough?" I'll tell you what I told him: that there are many different factors that affect a woman's ability to lubricate, with sexual excitement being only one of them.

The mucosal tissue of a woman's genitals is some of the most delicate tissue on her body, and even if she is totally wet and lubricated when you first start to stimulate her, once that area is exposed to air or condoms, it often dries out. So she can be totally turned on and still dry out. If the activity continues, she will start to feel a pulling and tearing and I can assure you that *that* feels none too nifty. The fact remains that some women, even when they are most aroused, don't always lubricate on cue. This biological fact reinforces the beauty of lubricants. And as I mentioned above, as with almost every facet of their anatomy and biology, women lubricate to varying degrees.

TIPS FOR USING LUBRICANTS

➤ During manual sex especially, put on lubricant by letting it drip through your fingers, hand in a downward trident shape (use three fingers). This works well for two reasons: (1) It warms up as it passes through your hand, and (2) the change in sensation from warm fingers to smoother, slicker palm can feel great.

➤ If you use saliva for lubricating your fingers, and you've had a glass of wine or a beer or two, remember that alcohol is a

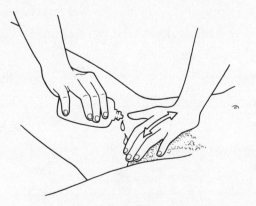

How to Administer Lubricant

natural desiccant for your system. It dries you up, so you may not have as much saliva as you normally would. Dreaded desert mouth at the wrong time.

➤ Putting oil inside a woman can give her a vaginal infection.

ONE-STOP SHOPPING

Most men don't enjoy shopping for products as much as women. From what I understand, gentlemen, you don't want to waste your time hanging out in the drugstore aisles or at an adult novelty store choosing among the huge array of lubricants on the market. What I have assembled for you is a list of the best and brightest lubricants, keeping in mind not only her pleasure but your own as well. For indeed, though she will enjoy the use of lubrication, *you* will reap the rewards.

There are many products to choose from, including those that are water-based, oil-based, flavored, nonflavored, scented, unscented, colored, clear, liquid, and gels. It can be a bit overwhelming. I asked my field researchers to investigate which lubricants felt and tasted the best. The results of our efforts are listed below, though this is by no means an exhaustive study.

SECRET FROM LOU'S ARCHIVES
Many women I know prefer colorless lubricants, as they won't stain the sheets or other materials.

FAVORITE LUBRICANTS
Again, this is not an exhaustive list, but you can use it as a general guide. (* means the product is colorless.)

➤ Astroglide.* The company uses "Second Only to Mother Nature" as its tag line, and our field researchers would have to agree it is the closest to our own natural intimate moisture. Astroglide is one of the most popular and easy-to-find brands of water-based personal lubricant. It has a slightly sweet taste and is odorless. You can buy it at your local drugstore and in many supermarkets as well. For anyone who wants the benefit of extra comfort during intercourse, but doesn't want to feel anything even the slightest bit unnatural, Astroglide is the lubricant of choice.

➤ Sensura/Sex Grease.* This is the water-based lubricant of choice for many connoisseurs. It is a clear thick liquid with a velvety texture that maintains a slick feel for a long time. The same product is marketed under two different names and packaged in two different ways. For the ladies it is called Sensura and bottled in pink. For the men it is called Sex Grease and bottled in black. This one beat out Astroglide for use during intercourse because of its slightly thicker, more velvety texture.

➤ Midnite Fire.* This lubricant comes in a small container with a snap-on lid. A woman from one of my seminars told me that whenever her husband wants her to come home "for a quickie," all he has to do is call her and snap open the lid of Midnite Fire over the phone. "It doesn't matter where I am—at my desk or in my car on the cell phone. When I hear that 'snap,' I am instantly wet!" Need I say more?

Midnite Fire is almost guaranteed to bring you lots of enjoyment. It not only comes in a variety of flavors, it also becomes very warm with gentle rubbing and even warmer when you blow on it following the rub. Not to worry, though, because the heat only builds to a certain level, so there is no risk of getting burned. It is the CO_2 in your breath that causes it to heat when you blow on it. Midnite Fire is a water-based lubricant, which is safe for application both internally and externally. Although it is billed as "The Hot Sensual Massage Lotion," it's really too thick to be used for a straight massage without adding water or another clear water-based lubricant. It feels especially erotic when applied to the nipples or inner thighs. Be aware if your lady has a predisposition for infections and test before going wild. It has also received rave reviews when used on the head of the penis and the testicles.

SECRET FROM LOU'S ARCHIVES

Beware of certain lubricants on the market that call themselves "body glides." Eros, Venus Millennium, and Platinum are newer products that are made of dimethicone (silicone) and carry no protective value and aren't water-soluble. Some even have a caution "flammable" or "for external use only" on the label. These are not only impractical; they may be dangerous if the silicone is absorbed by the body.

➤ Embrace. Truly one of the nicer tasting and feeling, this lubricant has a thick, velvety consistency similar to Sensura yet with a better taste for some. A favorite of those who want a lubricant to stay put when they apply it rather than having it run for lower elevations. It comes unflavored (which is slightly sweet) and in Strawberry and Lime Sherbet.

➤ Liquid Silk. The name describes it all. This creamy water-based British lubricant in a pump bottle contains no glycerin, so it doesn't get sticky and has become a favorite of field researchers. It is great for manual techniques and intercourse. It does, however, have a slightly bitter taste, which detracts from its use during oral sex.

➤ Maximus.* This is the clear version of Liquid Silk. It comes in a clear plastic pump bottle and is also a big favorite.

SECRET FROM LOU'S ARCHIVES

Be aware of inserting massage oil or any sugar-based product, including fruit, into your partner. These products can cause vaginal infections by altering the normal pH balance of the vaginal barrel.

TIPS FOR CHOOSING LUBRICANTS

➤ Know how sensitive you and your partner are to new products. Some women are so sensitive they can get bladder and vaginal infections from merely changing toilet tissue or soap.

➤ Always remember that oil and latex don't mix. Oil in any form is the mortal enemy of latex condoms, often causing them to break. Check the label of anything you're using, such as hand or massage lotions. If it says "oil" anywhere, you shouldn't use it as a lubricant with latex condoms. These lubricants are fine for manual sex, but if you're planning to continue on to intercourse using a condom, be sure to use a lubricant that is water-based.

➤ Always remember to read the label in its entirety. The big print alone can be misleading. If you see the word "oil" listed anywhere in the ingredients, chances are the product is not water-based.

➤ If you are sensitive or susceptible to irritation, watch out for the spermicide known as nonoxynol-9. As I discussed in Chapter Two, it can be extremely irritating to both men and women. This is the *only* manufactured spermicidal in the United States and it's the active ingredient in contraceptive foams/jellies, suppositories, film, and on condoms. Know what you're putting near or into your body and hers.

➤ Check to see if the product is okay for the genital area. Often the fine print on the package will say "for topical or cosmetic use" or "avoid contact with eyes." Also, nonoxynol-9 was introduced in the United States in 1920s as a cleaning solution for hospitals. Translation: it's a detergent. Can you imagine rubbing a detergent on your lady down there? This will give her pain, not pleasure.

➤ Remember that your lady is much more at risk for irritation and infection than you are. She is the receptive partner, and the products that you choose typically remain inside her.

It's about time we consumers hit the manufacturers of these products where it hurts—their bottom line. If you're reading this book, read *their* labels. If the bottle's back label in teensy-weensy print says "for topical cosmetic use only," what does that mean? And when they say "for external use only"? Hmmmm, I'll let you be the judge. Manufacturers also assume they can get away with dangerous or hurtful products, such as nonoxynol-9 and silicone, which can cause an allergic reaction or irritation. The only way they will stop producing them is if you stop buying them.

Positions

There are four main positions for manual play, and each position has moves best-suited to that position. As with any new idea or technique, use the suggestions below to add to or incorporate into what you already do. You may want to refer to the diagrams so that you and your lady will get the full benefit. Like dance steps, however, it's hard to know how to move until you actually see how it's done. In all of these positions, the man can maintain good body contact, which is key.

SECRET FROM LOU'S ARCHIVES

For all moves, start with a big motion, go to a smaller, more concentrated motion, and build from slow to quick tempo. Moving too quickly and firmly may numb or hurt her. Most women are not ready for that kind of instant intensity. Let the intensity build.

THE CLASSICS—POSITIONS 1 AND 5

These are probably the easiest and simplest positions to initiate manual stimulation of the lady and yet they are also the ones with the most bad habits. One woman in a seminar said, "If he did that 'staying in one spot right on top of my clit' for a second longer, I thought I would have to kill him." Another woman added, "Where are the directions that call for 'find it and rub furiously'?"

One of the reasons these popular positions have garnered bad habits comes from the fact that you've been fed a bill of goods by the adult porn industry through its videos and magazines. Their goal is to sell. They are not thinking of your personal pleasure, and they are certainly not think-

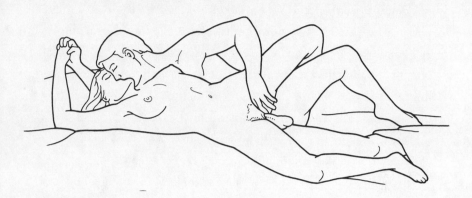

Position #1

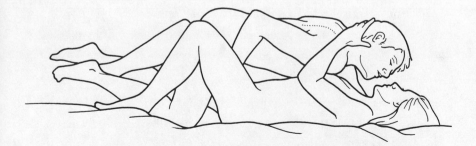

Position #5

ing about what pleases women. They are focusing on action, whether or not the action works. In real life, intense rubbing too soon or at all is often a sure way to cause your partner discomfort, not pleasure.

Gentlemen, the good news is that you can easily learn how to please your partner by simply adjusting the motion of your fingers and hand, your tempo, and the degree of pressure. After applying lubricant or moistening with saliva, you can use your fingers or the entire palm of your hand in a circular motion to (1) evenly spread the lubricant and (2) use a broader overall motion to warm things up in this area. It's best to start with the broad strokes and reduce the area of stimulation as sensation builds.

In both of these positions, it's a good idea to rest the heel of your hand (and the wrist) on her pubis mons, the area where the pubic hair starts, and gently apply pressure. You should feel the pubic bone underneath the base of your wrist. This will also help stabilize your wrist and arm. In other words, keeping your arm and hand in the air will tire you out more quickly and affect the overall fine-motion mobility of your fingers. With your wrist anchored, you can deliver more of the gentle circles and back-and-forth motions that women prefer.

These are also the manual positions that lend themselves best to kissing and snuggling. You can also use the index and middle fingers in a straight up-and-down and/or circular motion with the clitoral ridge and tip between the two of them. Often a woman uses this technique to stimulate herself. You can also use the palm of your hand.

If your penis is inside of her while you are touching her, try pulsing your PC muscle to make your penis pump. One woman remarked, "He does this penis-lifting thing when he is in me from behind that feels so good. It makes me all stretched and full of him." A male seminar attendee noted that "most women respond to this move by tightening inside, while the man moves his fingers back and forth."

IT TAKES 3.

This move will work best if you are behind her or on top of her. To start, you use three fingers held together to curve over the inner and outer lips. Keep your index finger and fourth finger on the outer edges of her outer labia while your middle finger is positioned on top of the entire clitoral ridge and bud. The benefit of starting with all three fingers is you don't shock the clitoris by going straight to it. Rather, you

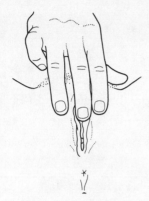

It Takes 3, Step 1

It Takes 3, Step 2

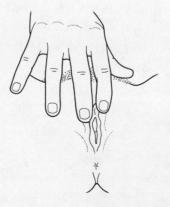

It Takes 3, Step 3

are building sensation around it. And because your hand is shielding her from airflow, your partner will feel the heat from your hand more directly and will stay wetter.

Now maintain a slow up-and-down or circular motion (consider outlining the alphabet if you need some inspiration for how to move your fingers). Then subtly slip the middle finger inside the vagina. Finally, with your index and middle fingers together, do a short range of motion over the clitoral ridge, moving from front to back, with a gentle squeeze, or a pulse up and down.

POSITION #2

This is a position chosen by men who love their lady's derriere. One man, a marketing executive from Portland, Oregon, said, "I love the roundness and feel of her ass and being able to play with her and smell her sex at the same time." This position also allows good access to her breasts. In this position, the man can use his thumb most effectively by inserting it into the vagina and doing a circular motion. Because the thumb is so much stronger than the fingers, it is the natural choice for long-term stimulation. This is also a great position for exploring G-spot sensation. Try using a curving pressure-stroke with middle and index finger on the front wall of her vagina. The G-spot will be felt more clearly, the more aroused she becomes. And if your partner likes anal play, this is a good way to initiate it.

Even before you get to the smaller action zone, you can build sensation over the back of her thighs, back of her knees, and the small of her back. Consider starting with a flat hand and finger so you can massage the greatest area. Then you can shrink down the area of stimulation by shifting the motions to your fingertips. And if she likes, you can shrink the motion even more by concentrating on the clitoral ridge and bud. Most men have said that bent index and middle fingers held together work best here, with the clitoral ridge cradled lengthwise between the two fingers. And remember to use your free hand to its greatest advantage by letting it roam around!

POSITION #3

The beauty of this position is that the woman can remain in very close contact with you and "melt" into your body. This is a favorite of those who like to watch and talk. In this position there are a number of technique options; however, it should go without saying, incorporate any of you and your partner's favored moves.

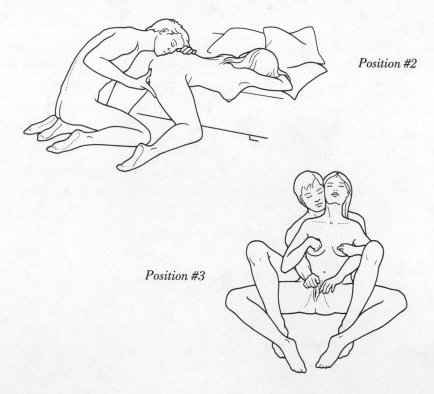

Position #2

Position #3

JR. DREIDEL (AKA MINI-FIRE STARTER).

This is a move in which she will truly appreciate your finesse. Just as generations of Jewish children do during Hanukkah, you will imi-

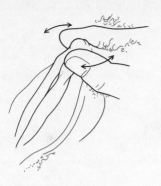

Jr. Dreidel

tate this spinning motion with your thumb to the absolute delight of your partner. Apply a touch of lubricant on your thumb and forefinger and use a gentle rotating motion. Be sure to use gentle pressure to start. This move will be easier for women with a larger clitoris. As with any move, make sure you ask her if she'd like to try this.

DOUBLE DUTY.

In this variation of the #3 position, the man's arms are on either side of the woman. He can use a strong, upward stroke, starting with the inside of the thighs and working toward the genitals. The idea behind this move is to relax her so she can "melt" into your body. As one woman said, "I feel so safe when we do this, even though I am totally exposed." You can create more buildup and sensation through her entire genital and pelvic area.

Double Duty

TOURING THE DANCE FLOOR.

This move requires a very light circular touch around the clitoris and labia. Start with simply tracing the outline of her genitals and then do the same move while gen-tly pulling the lips. The pulling move is a subtle way to heighten tension and builds sensation be-cause stretched skin tends to have greater feeling. Sometimes couples will incorporate an ice cube here. However, it's best to use it sparingly at first and just on the outside for about ten to twenty seconds. One woman said, "My

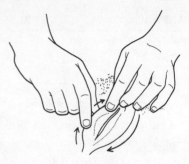

Touring the Dance Floor

husband did it once and I almost went through the ceiling. The cold was cold, but when he went down on me after with his mouth, he never felt so hot. The difference in temperature is what made it so awesome." A male seminar attendee remarked that this move was "very successful. It encourages taking your time." Some women, however, will not like this cold sensation, so don't surprise her.

Y-KNOT.

Spread the labia with two fingers of one hand, and with your other hand on top, position the middle finger, or two together, to massage the clitoris in a circular and/or up-and-down motion. This move is great in that it doesn't tire your hands. She also has a nice "big" feeling when your hands are covering her, instead of just a finger. You can also cover a greater area. You may want to try coming down on top: insert one or two fingers inside and curve them in and out of the vagina.

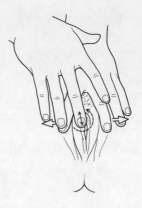
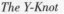

The Y-Knot

POSITION #4

This position is ideal for those times when a lady needs to feel she is "on her own." Some couples prefer the leg over the shoulder as a way to stay in contact while she concentrates on what you're doing. This provides a better view and it is easier on your back when you are at a

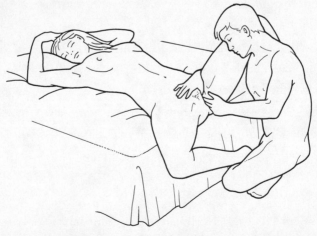

Position #4

lower level—consider stairs covered with pillows as an option. The lady can cover her tummy with sheets, should she get chilled.

THE WORLD IS YOUR OYSTER.

This move is best in the #4 position for two reasons: (1) There is more range of motion for you, and (2) you can concentrate on her while she concentrates on what you're doing. You will quite literally be touching her whole genital area as if it were soft, delicate clay and you are in the stages of final shaping and molding. Have lubricant handy, since this position and move require her to be quite spread open. This is another place to watch those nails. It's a slow buildup of sensation that will unravel her.

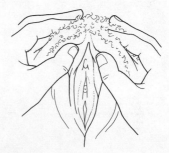

The World Is Your Oyster

THE SCULPTOR.

This move alternates between two placements—static, in which you stay in one place, and the dynamic, in which you change the hand orientation. The women in the seminars refer to both as the "take me home" moves.

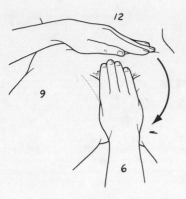

The Sculptor

Sculptor, Static Position—
The Big "C"

Static Position: Your hand is in the shape of a big "C." By orienting your thumb, imagine a clock over your partner's vulva and your thumb enters toward six o'clock and the side of the thumb curves up to twelve. There are a few critical things to remember with this: (1) With the web of your hand between thumb and forefinger and the inside knuckle area of your index finger, you will be creating sensation while you use the circular, rocking "C" motion; (2) the inside edge of your thumb can be putting pressure on the G-spot by maintaining an upward pressure, toward her belly button, on the upper vaginal wall; this sensation can be further heightened by (3) using your other hand to press down on her abdomen in the pubic hair. You should be able to feel the slight pressure of the side of your thumb through her abdomen. Also while using the rocking "C" motion, try spreading your "C" fingers and put the pressure on the mons pubis area. Many women enjoy pressure there while being stimulated.

Dynamic Position.

In the dynamic position, your thumb moves from the twelve o'clock position and, using a continuous motion, moves to each position of her internal clock (twelve to six). When you reach six o'clock, change and insert your index and middle fingers to complete the cycle back up to the twelve position. Use your free hand to apply a stretching pressure to the skin on her abdomen, and upward toward her belly button, to heighten sensation.

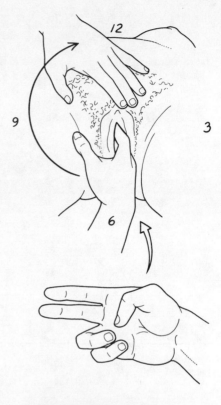

Sculptor, Dynamic Position—
After Six O'Clock

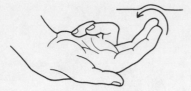

"Come Here" Motion

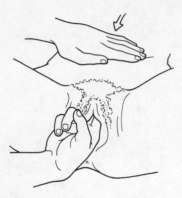

G-Man Position A

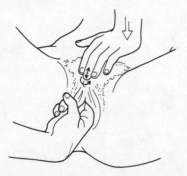

G-Man Position B

G-MAN.

The G-Man also has two hand-placement variations, A and B.

Position A: Insert your index and middle fingers and use a "come here" motion against her G-spot region. Remembering that the G-spot is above the vaginal wall, you can press on her abdomen to heighten the sensation for her.

Position B: It's important to remember that your top hand is not just supplying pressure. Remember these points: Use your middle finger or thumb to stimulate her clitoral area while the other hand's fingers are caressing her G-spot and the heel of your top hand is maintaining the pressure and stimulation.

FROG PRINCE.

Remember those swim lessons? You will be doing a frog kick stroke inside of her using your index and middle fingers. Your hand can be in either a vertical or a horizontal orientation. The idea behind this move is women's differing sensitivities in vaginal walls. The Shimmy can be done in combination with the Frog Prince. In this submove, you shimmy your two fingers in and out of her, so you can feel both sides of the vaginal walls.

Tips to Keep in Mind When Touching Her Genitals

➤ Avoid homing-pigeon fingers. Chances are, if she shifts her hips ever so slightly, that is *exactly* where she wants you to stay, so please do not go back to the spot she has just moved your fingers from.

➤ Cease and desist from the Dip-Test, which looks like this: kiss, kiss, kiss (the lips); tweak, tweak, tweak (the nipples); dip, dip, dip (between her legs). This is not considered relaxing or stimulating to most women.

➤ The poke between the legs and "Oh goodie, she's ready" makes women feel like they are operating parts. Solution: Pay attention to her breathing. The more relaxed a lady is, the deeper and more relaxed her breathing becomes. The change in her breathing will let you know the other mental "stuff" is melting away.

➤ A woman will start lubricating intravaginally within thirty seconds of being stimulated either mentally or physically. Some women naturally have lots of lubrication; it is very individualistic and also subject to the influence of how hydrated she is, if she is on medication, and where she is in her cycle, and that includes menopausal women as well.

➤ Avoid always going immediately to the action spots, such as her breasts and genitals. Remember, her skin is her largest sexual organ, so take full advantage of that. Linger all over her body and use your Swirl techniques.

Manual stimulation can lead anywhere, but many women love for it to be followed by a man's most intimate gesture: kissing her "down there" with his tongue. With that in mind, the next chapter will help illuminate the wondrous delights your tongue can deliver.

SIX

The Art of Tongue: Leading a Woman to Rapture

Rising Humidity

Your mouth can create many more sensations than any other part of your body. Ask most women and, if they're being honest, they will admit that what makes them hottest and come hardest is when a man can use his tongue well. If there is one story that your partners gratefully and ofttimes wistfully share in the seminars, it is about the man who can give her great oral sex. One woman said, "I love having him between my legs. There isn't anything that feels better." Another woman said, "I can't describe what he did, but it was phenomenal! I knew he loved women. He didn't care how much time it took. If there is one word to describe him, I would say perseverance. I must admit, his technique was legendary."

Another testament to the alluring power of your tongue comes from an advertising executive from Seattle, who said, "What makes [oral sex] so good is that it doesn't leave me feeling sore. When he goes down on me, his tongue and mouth are so hot and soft, it's both soothing and exciting."

Need I say more? Women respond to oral sex.

As you know by now, I am a firm believer that anything worth doing is worth doing well. Therefore, this chapter contains information that will not only make you a competent purveyor of oral treats but an expert who will bring a woman to her knees when she sees you licking your lips.

Now, I know some of you are uncomfortable with this whole subject. Indeed, some of you may actually avoid it altogether. And while you have every right in the world to refrain from doing what makes you uncomfortable, I will point out some of the reasons either you or your partner may feel hesitant to let go and enjoy the pleasures of oral sex. But if, after you've gone through this entire chapter, you still feel reluctant to give her oral sex, then you should be honest about it. In a gentle, kind way explain your feelings. Keep in mind, however, that your partner is especially vulnerable to the slightest rejection in this area. Women will take it personally if you don't handle it with kid gloves. Also remember that women know or sense when a man is not enjoying himself, and the last thing a woman wants is for you to do something you're not enjoying.

Part of the reason that some women feel uncomfortable about oral sex is that they carry around with them the feeling that their genitals are unclean or that men find oral sex distasteful. We can thank Madison Avenue and their clients for that charming legacy. It was the advertisers who developed the "need" for douching and reinforced negative or shameful feelings about female genitalia. To the contrary, as I've already stated, a healthy woman's genital area is one of the most self-cleansing and self-maintaining aspects of her body. Ironically, sexual intercourse is the number one reason behind most genital problems in women. Specifically, yeast and bladder infections and STDs result from having a foreign substance (semen) introduced into a woman's body. As you've seen in previous chapters, women can also suffer from problems in reaction to nonoxynol-9. As one of the top specialists in this area said, "Women who do not have sex have the most pristine vaginal canals."

But I have talked to women who say that they're afraid they smell and/or will taste bad. If a woman is clean and doesn't have infection, she should not smell or taste bad. Then again, it's very individualistic—she may just not smell good to you. However, if you pay attention to her scent, you may find it stimulating—this is, after all, the idea behind pheromones. Just as she is attracted to your male scent, so you are to hers.

Factors that will change your lover's taste:

➤ Vitamins
➤ Medication
➤ Diet
➤ Where she is in her cycle
➤ Infection
➤ Degree of hydration
➤ Spicy or heavily seasoned foods
➤ Alcohol, drugs, or tobacco

SECRET FROM LOU'S ARCHIVES

A pheromone is a substance that provides chemical means of communication between animals and certain insects, detected by smell. May affect development, reproduction, and behavior.

It's important for you and the women in your life to participate in tearing down some of the old myths having to do with oral sex being dirty or unnatural. Some men and women still believe this, and I feel they are missing out on one of the most pleasurable experiences two people can share and give one another. If it's so "unnatural," why do male animals invariably approach a female's genitals with their nose and mouth? It's up to you to release her inhibitions and your own. Chances are you both will find boundless pleasure in this activity.

In my countless seminars, women have shared with me that they often feel safer and more enthusiastic about oral sex if you refer to it in a nicer way. Sadly, many of our cultural references having to do with the female body are derisive or unpleasant. Here are some options that women report preferring: "eaten out," "going down on me," "cunnilingus," "giving me head," "dining out, "going south of the border." Phrases that are not liked include: "box lunch," "eating pussy," "bush burgers," and "muff diving."

SECRET FROM LOU'S ARCHIVE:
Not all women are able to orgasm with cunnilingus, just as not all men are able to orgasm with fellatio.

The majority of men who are great at this have learned from women—not from adult material or friends. Why? Because, as I've said before, the porn industry is inaccurate and insists on depicting cunnilingus as a long tongue pointed in the general direction of a woman's anatomy. Invariably, the tongue is not even close to the clitoris. Another problem some men have shared with me is they don't know their way around a woman's anatomy and feel they are "rooting around in the dark." This is perfectly understandable, and another reason why I included the guide to genitalia in the previous chapter. If you know that the clitoris is under a hood, for instance, then you'll know where to focus and why when it is stimulated it becomes engorged lifting under the hood.

Herein lies one of the great faux pas of oral sex: the "flicking" problem. Flicking directly on the clitoris, especially in the initial stage, is not stimulating for most women. Now, some women enjoy flicking, but not until they are already stimulated. It's better to start with a full, warm mouth on her, and then some flicking, and then back to full, warm mouth. One male seminar attendee suggests "leading up to her clitoris by stroking your tongue on her inner thighs, and working your way up to the pubic bone, where you put on a bit of pressure."

Three things are bound to happen with flicking: (1) Your tongue dries out; (2) she dries out; and (3) your dry tongue pulls on her clitoris—not pleasurable. As one woman aptly put it, "What is it with those flickers? Why do they stay so far away? Are they afraid to come close? Tell them to suck on us the way they want us to suck on them," she said, muttering as she walked out of the room.

But inaccurate information promoting flicking is indeed out there. A passage in a recently published book compiled by the editors of *Men's Health* magazine says men should "flick" a woman's clit and not touch the lips with your lips. This is absolutely wrong! No wonder men feel frustrated and women feel disappointed! The author then goes on to say that "you can't smother the clitoris with your lips or you'll deaden the sensation." In fact, the opposite is true—the clitoris does like to have isolated touch (with tongue), but the whole area responds to gentle sucking and pressure. The key is in knowing (which may require asking) what your lover enjoys. And, gentlemen, she may not know her own body; again as a compassionate lover, it's partly your role to help her understand her own body.

Maintenance and Hygiene

The best and most effective way for a woman to maintain herself in "dining condition" is regular bathing and cleaning of the genital area. If you are concerned that she is not fresh as a daisy, perhaps you can suggest taking a shower together. One woman from a seminar told me that her boyfriend lays her on the bed, inches up her dress, and slowly washes her with a warm, wet washcloth. When he's finished, they are both totally turned on: She is completely aroused and he is, too. As she explains, "I feel like he is completely embracing of me, which just gets me so hot."

If you try the washcloth method, remember not to use soap. The pH in soap is incompatible with the natural pH of a woman's body. The soap will upset the natural acid balance that keeps the vaginal environment stable and braced to fight off foreign, infecting substances. The lemony tartness of a woman's natural lubrication is from the more acidic lubrication, the lactic acid. Vitamins will also change (usually for the worse) her taste. While we are on this subject, if you are concerned about how to let your lady know her smell or taste is strong, try telling her about the last time she tasted *good*, after eating such foods as fruit.

SECRET FROM LOU'S ARCHIVES

If your partner shaves her pubic hair, be careful of regrowth during oral sex and intercourse. Stubble could be abrasive for you.

THE TRIANGLE DEBATE

Some men love a lot of pubic hair. The wife of a major television star said, "He'd love it if I never shaved my legs, armpits, or bush. I'm the one who prefers it off." For other men, less hair is definitely more. You may want to know that the current fashion trends do require some pretty close manicuring of women's pubic hair: (1) naked lips, (2) clean thong (area between buttocks cheeks), and (3) a small triangle or "runway" of hair. Some women will have special-event waxings done—hearts for Valentine's Day and shamrocks for St. Patrick's Day are two rather vivid examples. However, these designs do require skilled estheticians. One woman from a seminar told me about having her pubic hair dusted with gold powder (to match her lingerie) for a special occasion. After a night of complete enjoyment, her boyfriend left the next morning to play his regular basketball game. As he walked on the court, his teammates looked at him and asked, "What the f— is all over your face?" You guessed—her gold dust. So if she dapples, just check yourself in the mirror before going out in public.

SECRET FROM LOU'S ARCHIVES

If you are worried about stray hairs in your mouth, do a stroking move with your hand through her pubic hair. She will take it as a caressing move, when in actuality, you are grooming her and removing loose hairs.

While we are on the subject of her hair, I'd like to address *your* facial hair. Make sure that after shaving, you are smooth enough to approach her. Rub the inside of your wrist on your beard, particularly just below your lower lip. If you feel anything scratchy, so will she. One woman, who has particularly sensitive skin, told me of being left with a rash on the inside of her thigh—ouch! Short mustaches and goatees can be the most abrasive, so longer hair (beards) is generally better.

The significance of your hair is best captured by this anecdote from one of my seminars. In a group of thirty-five men, I asked the three men with facial hair if they ever used their beards as a tool in oral foreplay. (Please note that these men did not know each other.) The three men shyly looked at each other and then smiled. In unison, all three nodded yes. Then one of them, a big trucker, announced as he stroked his very full beard, "Hell, I even use hair conditioner on mine so it's nice and soft."

But as a standard policy, ask her what *she* prefers.

SECRET FROM LOU'S ARCHIVES

In French, a woman's personal scent is referred to as her "cassolette."

Lifting the Clitoral Hood

For those ladies who enjoy and prefer direct clitoral stimulation, you will need to lift the prepuce, or clitoral hood (akin to the foreskin in a man). Here are some tips.

Option #1: Using the index and middle fingers of both hands, put upward pressure on the inside of the outer labia and lift the entire area. The best positions for this are the Classic (oral), SOMF, and Chair Therapy.

Option #2: The woman's legs must be in a "V" with her feet on a flat surface. You are between her legs and have one arm under and around her thigh. With a flat hand on her pubic hair, use a firm, upward pressure toward her head. Again, this will move everything up and create a more taut, open area for your mouth.

Option #3: If she is comfortable doing so, ask your partner to hold herself open. She might get a better hold on the slippery surface of the skin if she wears those little white cotton gloves—the type women wore in the 1950s. Of course, she may feel silly doing this, so it's up to both of you to decide.

Positions

A quick note before I describe the best positions for oral sex. I'd like to share what some men recommend as great ways to practice tongue technique.

1. Eat an ice cream cone. Just think about it: The upward, elongating tongue strokes are quite similar to what you would use on her. For more subtle moves, try eating Jell-O or pudding straight out of the container with no spoon.
2. To perfect your tongue finesse (and as Whoopi Goldberg suggested in her comedy routine), hold a Life Saver at the front of your mouth in the flat position either between your lips and gum or just inside your teeth. Using tiny tongue motions, "eat" or dissolve the Life Saver from inside out. Like great oral sex, this takes time, patience, and a strong, nimble tongue.

That said, we're ready to move on to the positions. Essentially, there are five positions, with each position containing subpositions or variations on the main theme.

THE CLASSICS

In the following seven illustrations, you'll see the standard position of the man between the woman's legs, with his mouth attached to her genitals. And although these seven positions all belong to the same "family," each has its own variation on the theme. As a rule, it's best to have pillows under her hips and under your chest. This allows for a better range of motion for you and positions her hips so she can be spread more openly. It also saves you from abrading the underside of your tongue on your teeth.

Straight-On: (Positions A and B) These two positions allow for good upward stroking, lifting the clitoral hood. In A and B, the woman can adjust how open she is by holding her thighs open. She can also use her hands (perhaps in those white gloves) to pull up on the outer labia to assist her partner. In these two positions, you can easily incorporate the "hand assist" (see page 156), using the thumb to stroke the anus or inserting one or two fingers into the vagina to put pressure on the bottom of the introitus, the vaginal opening. Keep your fingers in slow motion and use circular movements.

T-Cross: This is a good stroke for ladies who are more sensitive on one side of their clitoris than the other. The gentleman can alternate between a broad stroke and a pointy one, circling the clitoral bud.

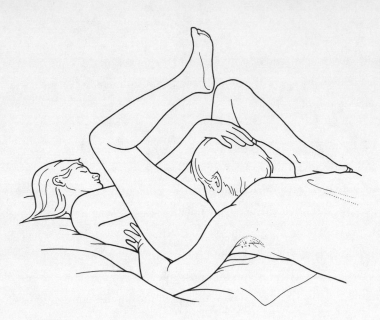

Straight On, Position A

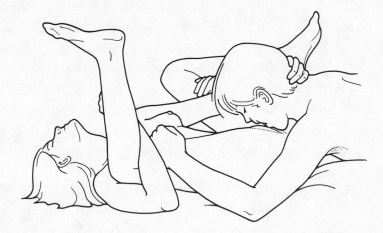

Straight On, Position B

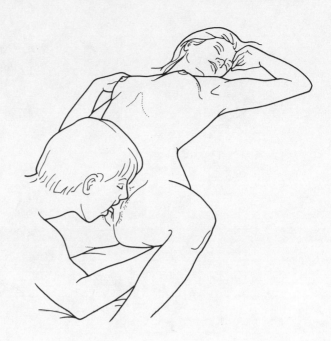

T-Cross

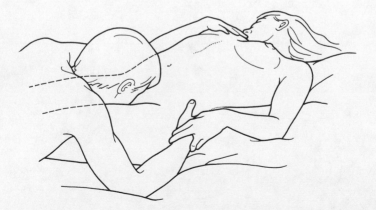

Legs Together

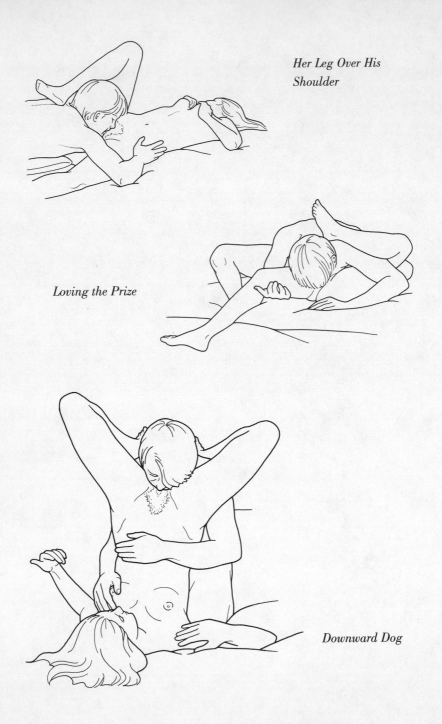

Her Leg Over His Shoulder

Loving the Prize

Downward Dog

Legs Together: This is a good starting point and often the best for a woman with a hypersensitive clitoris, who cannot tolerate strong direct contact.

Her Leg over His Shoulder: Have her place one leg over your shoulder, and with a slight twist of her hips, you will be able to reach the right spot. Women have said they feel more connected in this position. Again, use an upward stroking motion.

Loving the Prize: This is an ideal position for staying more connected to each other. Using a downward stroke, the man is able to relax the angle of his head, relieving his neck muscles.

Downward Dog: This is a play on the downward-facing-dog yoga position. For most couples, this is more of a novelty position, but it does allow for a good view of your partner. And some women enjoy feeling their partner holding them tightly around the middle and playing with their breasts. Again, use an upward stroking motion and be sure not to put too much weight on her.

SECRET FROM LOU'S ARCHIVES

When some women orgasm via oral sex, there is a change in consistency of lubrication. One man said, "She got thicker and there was more of it."

SIDE BY SIDE AND THE 69

A transition position for oral sex, the Side by Side and the 69 require tremendous concentration. One woman reported, "I couldn't give head and receive it at the same time. It was too much like that

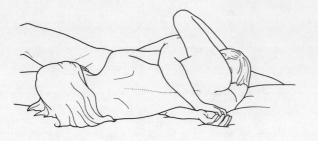

Side by Side

69

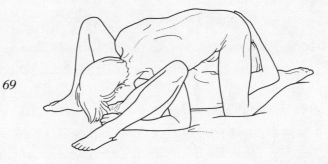

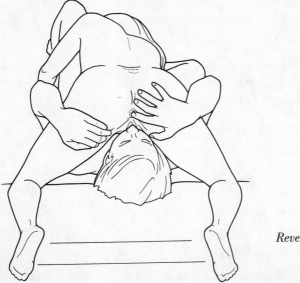

Reverse 69

tummy-rubbing, head-patting move. I like to warm up in this position and then switch positions."

Using a downward stroking motion, this is for more sensitive ladies. Make sure there is a lot of saliva so she won't dry out. While you're busy, she can be sucking on your penis or testicles. It's a relaxing position for your neck, too.

On your side, you can cushion your head on her thigh. As one man put it, "My tongue stays more moist, saliva pools in my mouth, so I can taste her more." You can also reach around and play with her buttocks and anus.

With the woman over the top of the man, you can relax every part of your body—except your tongue. Use a downward stroking motion. This is ideal for partners who enjoy oral/manual anal play.

THE ARCH

This is another novelty position that requires the man sitting up, with his partner on top. She then stays in place by locking her ankles behind his head while her thighs rest on his shoulders. Some women enjoy the blood rush to the head when they go horizontal again.

SOMF (SIT ON MY FACE)
AND HOVERING BUTTERFLY

These positions are two of the easiest for the lady to control the motion. In both the forward-facing Hovering Butterfly toward his head and the away-facing SOMF, she can adjust the pressure and speed as she chooses.

SOMF. Your head and neck should be supported by a pillow—not only for comfort but so you have some vertical give

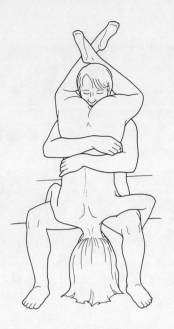

The Arch

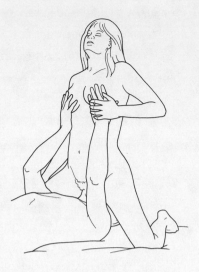

Sit on My Face

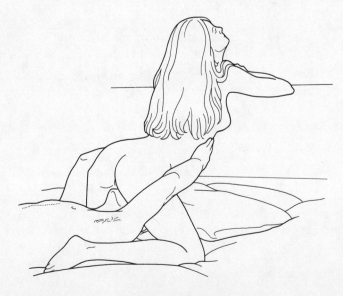

Hovering Butterfly

in the stroking area. You can easily play with her breasts and use your hands to open her more. Use both downward and upward stroking motions and lots of suction. This way she is able to concentrate on her own pleasure, as she can't do anything to you.

Hovering Butterfly. This is a ladies' favorite for a number of reasons. She can rest on something and feel very much in control while her partner is doing her. Use a good upward stroking motion. An optional move is to cover yourself from the waist down while she faces your feet.

REAR APPROACH

This position is a favorite of men who love a woman's buttocks. It requires a shallower stroking motion, however, and if you decide to go into any anal play, remember not to go back to her vulvar area, as you don't want to transfer fluids or organisms from one area to the other. Since the naturally occurring organisms of the anal (both yours and hers) and vaginal areas differ, you risk upsetting her natural vaginal environment, which may then cause her to get vaginal or bladder infections.

You have limited access to everything here, but it is a good starting position. You may have to crook your neck quite severely. One woman's comment was, "I love when my husband does this. It's so animal—it turns me on." In this position, with her shoulders dropped,

> ### SECRET FROM LOU'S ARCHIVES
> Don't go anywhere with your tongue or finger after you've gone near the anus; you risk introducing foreign organisms that can then cause infection.

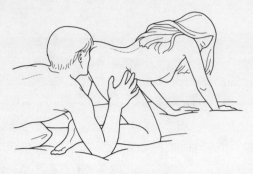

Rear Approach

Chair Therapy

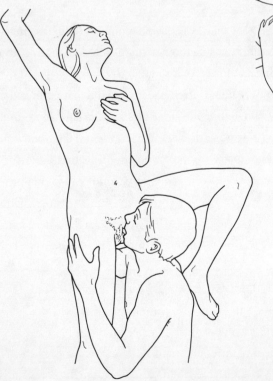

Stand and Deliver

she can help pull herself open with her hands and open up the entire area.

CHAIR THERAPY AND STANDING UP

These two positions lend themselves to activity outside of the bedroom.

Chair Therapy: Whether she's perched on a countertop or a sofa, the lady has a great view and the man a position he can maintain for an extended period without getting a sore neck. The lady can stay connected by holding his head, though some men claim this feels like being "grabbed behind the ears and steered like a boat." If she sits or reclines on a table and you're on a chair, the benefits are obvious: You're totally comfortable and can concentrate on the job at hand, so to speak, using "hand assist" moves to pleasure her more.

Stand and Deliver: Another acrobatic position, often used in the shower or while getting dressed or undressed. Use an upward stroking here. This position is a terrific way to increase what I call the fun factor of great sex. Anytime you introduce a new position, new move, or new item, you are increasing the spirit of adventure, which will in turn make you both feel more spontaneous, playful, and excited. Unfortunately, the only downside is the gentleman sometimes gets a bad crick in his neck.

Special Moves

Strumming the Frenulum. Technically, the frenulum is a skin attachment point. Men have one on the head of their penis, and women have it on the top of their vulvar/clitoral area. To please a woman here, use the undersurface of your tongue (it's much smoother) with a quick side-to-side stroke. Your tongue will be curved up close to your upper lip.

The Elevator. Use the top surface of your tongue in an upward stroke and use the undersurface on the downward stroke.

Doing Your ABCs. I believe it was the late Sam Kinison, a raunchy-style comedian, who brought this technique to fame. Alternate tongue moves that are easy to remember write the letters of your alphabet. To make it even more exciting, try enlarging the font and italicizing. You may want to ask her to hold herself more open for you.

Mr. Hoover. This is all about suction, which most women really enjoy. Have her suck on your fingers to show you how she likes to be stimulated.

Cradle and Diamond Tip. Suck on the clitoral bud and use the tip of your tongue to stimulate it while you are creating suction pressure with your pursed lips.

Ice Cubes. Some women love this, but others don't like the cold sensation at all.

The Picasso. Use your tongue to create a line drawing all over her body, using her clitoris as a launching point. This is also where you can show her what she tastes like by surfacing and kissing her.

Some General Tips from the Field

> One woman finally found a way to tell her partner how she liked to be licked. "I told him to kiss my pussy the same way he kisses my lips—big, soft, wet, and warm. Then I told him

that I wanted him to suck on my clit the same way he sucks on my tongue."

➤ When women say "That's great," or "There," men often speed up, or increase the pressure. This ends up rushing her, which will totally cut the legs out from under her "slow buildup." At the risk of repeating myself, you need to let the lady relax into the sensations—that's how things really build. On the other hand, when she says "more," by all means stay with that motion.

➤ Men who are best at this use their entire face, and say they resemble a glazed donut when they're through. If your tongue gets tired, use your nose and chin to execute your moves.

➤ Men have shared that some women like when you put pressure on their mons pubis with your nose.

➤ While you are using your tongue to stimulate her clitoris, consider using firm, steady pressure on the urethral area, just below the clitoris, with the front of your chin. Also, some women enjoy chin pressure on the base of the introitus.

➤ A woman who was extremely sensitive to touch directly on her clitoris wore silk panties when her husband went down on her. She would still be highly stimulated through the silk, but not too much. After all, silk isn't waterproof.

➤ The slower you go, the faster you'll get there—honest. "Sometimes he's at speed 4, and I haven't even gotten into gear." In order for a woman to orgasm, she needs to have a buildup of tension. The speed of movement should build slowly and gradually. Then, as she begins to approach orgasm, speed up and direct your tongue more intensely.

➤ During oral sex, women tend to feel that a man is far away. You may want to consider a more body-contacting position (see Loving the Prize in the Classic position).

➤ Some women like you to move your tongue in small, repetitive motion, whereas other women want variety. She may want you to use your tongue in broad, general strokes in the beginning, and then as she becomes excited, she may want you to zero in on her clitoris and concentrate on that spot. Check in with her and ask if she would like you to change the motions of your tongue.

➤ Keep in mind that for most women, especially if oral sex is the first move of foreplay, it's going to take longer than you think to orgasm. Some women take fifteen minutes; others take up to a half hour. It depends on many variables, including how relaxed and comfortable she is.

➤ One of the best ways a man can tell if a woman is relaxing and getting more excited is through her breath: It will change, slow, and deepen. As she gets closer to orgasm, use her breathing as a guide to quicken, slow, or change the degree of movement of your tongue and mouth. Another indication of her arousal may be if she arches her back and goes up on her shoulders.

➤ Some women get overstimulated during oral sex. If that's the case, you need to either vary the intensity or range of your tongue's movement or orally caress another part of her body and give her genitals a rest. Often if you return your tongue to her clitoris or labia after a short rest, she will still be aroused, but still able to have an orgasm.

➤ Some women who feel they are not going to orgasm during or from oral stimulation can experience anxiety. Try to help your partner, letting her know that it's perfectly okay not to orgasm.

SECRET FROM LOU'S ARCHIVES

Some women like the sensation of a man "humming" on them.

TROUBLESHOOTING

We all know, women included, that pleasing her orally requires some slight contortions of your head and body. Here are some solutions:

KNOTS IN THE NECK SOLUTIONS

1. Pillows, pillows, pillows. Use them, especially if you're on a bed, under her hips and/or under your chest. (In Hovering Butterfly, use a pillow under your head.)
2. Use the wag. This is an action of wagging your head like you are signaling "no" while keeping your tongue extended and in contact with her.

YOUR TONGUE GETS TIRED

1. If your tongue gets tired, curve it up against the outside of your upper lip. This way, you can relax your tongue and not break the sensation of softness and heat she is enjoying.

2. There are two surfaces on your tongue—top and bottom. If your tongue tires in a side stroking motion, relax with a big upward stroke with the top surface. Then use the soft underside of your tongue on the downward stroke.

USE THE HAND ASSIST

1. The hands and mouth work in concert. While your mouth is on her, use your fingers, too. Specifically, try sliding your thumb around the perineal or anal area.
2. Pressure the bottom of the introitus area, inside the vagina. If a woman is on her back and you are looking at her genitals, the introitus is the vaginal opening. Using your thumb or chin, pressure the bottom of this entry within the first two inches. Some women become very aroused.
3. Keep a hand under your chin. This is a multitasking move. Not only can you support your chin in the crest of your thumb and forefinger, you can also use the second joint at the front of your index finger to continue the stroking motion while your tongue takes a break. By the time you need to do this, there should be enough lubrication from her to avoid any dryness.

FACIAL HAIR SNAFUS

1. Make sure you shave yourself like a baby's butt, especially around your mouth and right under your lower lip. Test on the inside of your wrist. If you feel it, so will she, and for her it will feel like sandpaper.
2. I have learned that a lot more men are enjoying the pleasures of trimming or shaving their partner's pubic hair. You may

want to try it as a form of erotic foreplay. Men have also said it's neater and tidier, which they like.

Since so many women enjoy oral stimulation in order to orgasm, indulge her. Your tongue is a magical instrument, and your lover will be eternally grateful if you learn to use it as openly, generously, and playfully as you like. Remember, your tongue on her is a sign of your total acceptance of her.

—— • ——

SEVEN

Assembling (and Expanding) Your Tool Chest

You're Never Too Old for Toys

Do you know how many more men and women use sex toys today than a decade ago? The numbers will probably surprise you. According to two adult novelty manufacturers, the market has increased tenfold over the past ten years, becoming a $500-million retail business. Experts attribute such a marked increase in the use of sex toys to a couple of reasons. In general, one manufacturer explains that "there is less stigma" attached to toys than there used to be. Furthermore, couples feel there is more openness in marriages to try new things. The manufacturer said, "Men and women are feeling pressure to remain monogamous and be safer about sex. As a result, they are looking for inventive ways to spice up their sex lives." Long associated with subjects less than respectful, sex toys and other "adult toys" have come out of the proverbial closet. Clear evidence of this turnaround is the fact that some of our grandmothers and great-grandmothers were using vibrators, showing us that they were a lot more progressive in this area than we had any idea. So keep reading.

First let me say that these products are not meant to replace passionate, connecting lovemaking. It is a given that the majority of women in the ladies' seminars genuinely like men and want to be around men. (And the same can be said of the men in the men's seminars, regarding women.) This is true despite the fact that we may not necessarily understand men at all times. So again, toys are not meant to replace either partner. They are simply meant to enhance our sexual experience and add a bit of fun to our sex lives. As one man, a triathlete from Los Angeles, said, "I'm just going to design my own tool belt. I'll slap a bottle of lubricant on one side and a vibrator on the other. Then I'll be all set."

If you or your partner is unfamiliar with sex toys, then be respectful and courteous in how you suggest introducing them into your relationship. Women can be shy and may think the toys are a sign of your dissatisfaction. If that thought gets into her head, she may withdraw from the toys *and* you. After her boyfriend suggested they play with a vibrator, one woman said, "I went straight to 'I'm not adequate enough as a lover.' And it wasn't until he told me he got them because he thought we'd have fun that I realized how off-base I was." Another woman said, "What started out as a joke gift led us to look at other toys that are now a really fun part of what we do together."

She needs to know from you that toys are something you want to share with her. You need to emphasize that it's the freedom in your relationship that enables you both to experiment and loosen the boundaries of the tried-and-true. It's the icing on the cake—and it's not all the time.

Keep in mind, too, that neither of you is expected to know how to already use these items. Look at some of them and you may think, "What on earth is it?" Every industry has its own trade show, and the one I attend happens to be the semiannual ANME (Adult Novelty Manufacturers Expo); in essence, it's a trade show for sex toys. I can assure you there are times that I see a product and think, "What were they thinking?!" (Some of these products are not really intended to work; they are simply made to sell.) Then there are other times when a product seems interesting and I hand it over to my field researchers, who then try it and give me feedback. The diagrams and directions below will shed some light on those toys that received the highest praise. You need to give both of you the permission to introduce something new and have some fun with toys—after all, isn't bringing something new a natural part of intimacy?

Vibrators

So we get things straight, a vibrator is any imaginatively shaped instrument that has the ability to vibrate and can be used to stimulate a woman or a man. Generally, vibrators are in the shape of a penis and are made of a hard, plasticlike material (in order to contain the battery or electrical motor component). For those of you who are even the smallest bit reluctant to chart this new territory, let me repeat myself: Vibrators can never replace the physical you. These items, like other sex toys, only enhance a woman's pleasure with you and may even help relax her in unexpected ways. Vibrators are invariably the fastest and quickest masturbatory route. When used together with your partner, they can make sex between you and her even more uninhibited and fun.

Let me dispel another myth: Vibrators should not desensitize her to your touch or penetration, nor do they pose competition. In the same way that most men learn how to orgasm most quickly by masturbating, some women learn how to climax through vibrators. Yet there is a big difference between her vibrator and your hands, fingers, tongue, and penis. Having said that, if this is the only way a woman can climax, then please indulge her—a vibrator can create much more intense stimulation than her hand or your body can. There are essentially three reasons that vibrators make it easy for a woman to orgasm. One is the intensity of the vibration. Another is that when a woman uses it, she is typically by herself and therefore more relaxed. The third reason is that she knows exactly where to place the stimulation and at what intensity.

Some women, however, after longtime continuous use, may have become more reliant than they think, and part of your job (as her helpful sexual playmate) is to help wean her of her dependence.

You should be aware that there are new "silent" vibrators, so-called because of their very high frequency. These vibrators have been reported to numb. A man I know who uses vibrators with his wife tried one of these silent types on his scrotum through his jeans. Five minutes after he'd stopped using it, the whole area began to throb and hurt from the overstimulation. Perhaps this is when your mother's advice to do "everything in moderation, dear" comes into play.

SECRET FROM LOU'S ARCHIVES

Not all women like or use vibrators. One woman said, "It was too noisy and distracting. I felt like my orgasm had been pulled out of me. It cut off the buildup."

You may find it interesting that the electric vibrator was invented in the late nineteenth century by American doctors as a labor-saving device for their treatment of "female disorders." Women would go to their doctors to receive "treatment" for their "nerves." The treatment entailed manual stimulation by the doctor until the women orgasmed and were relieved from the built-up tension. The practice went on until a fatigued doctor invented a mini-appliance (otherwise known as a vibrator) to assist him in the procedure. Patient visits suddenly became quicker and easier on the doctors, and vibrators were soon marketed as home appliances in women's magazines and mail-order catalogs, where they were hyped as cure-alls for headaches, asthma, "fading beauty," and even tuberculosis! Vibrators experienced a fall from grace, however, when they started showing up in stag films and their obvious sexual association could no longer be denied.

The majority of men think that vibrators are only for women. This is yet another myth. I have spoken to a number of men who have discovered the joys of vibration. Essentially, you should feel free to use them in any way that makes sense, is safe and clean, and doesn't hurt.

Women who use vibrators tend to fall into one of two camps. Either they prefer the intense clitoral stimulation of the small-headed vibrators, or they prefer the larger-headed vibrators (such as the Hitachi Magic Wand), which give vibration over a larger area. But you never know how you may sexually surprise her, so use your imagination!

TYPES OF VIBRATORS

There are umpteen styles, sizes, shapes, and colors of vibrators. They are powered by one of two sources—electricity or batteries. They are travel-size or made to leave at home. Some have smooth surfaces, while others come with ridges—just like some potato chips. Other vibrators come with protruding attachments to stimulate more than one area at a time (see the Rabbit Pearl below). The following sampling (the favorites among the women and men in my seminars) should give you a heads-up to begin your search for the perfect vibrator for you.

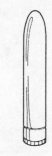

Wand Style

- ➤ "Wand style" describes the shape of the vibrator and is therefore the most recognizable of the various styles. It is usually made of hard plastic and powered by batteries.
- ➤ Coil-operated vibrators were originally designed for sore neck and muscle massage. Often electrically powered, they tend to be larger and stronger than the wand style. Some older coil-operated vibrators strap onto the back of your hand for legitimate massage work. They come with various attachments and are the easiest to disguise as being for another purpose.
- ➤ Finger Tip and Remote-controlled vibrators are distinctive for their ability to create a surprise effect. Manufacturers finally have some that work!

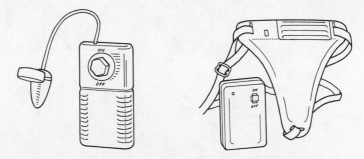

Finger Tip Style   *Remote Style*

➤ Waterproof vibrators are capable of accompanying you and your partner in the shower! They range in size from small handheld ones to larger, soft, foam-covered balls four inches in diameter that can be used over the entire body.

SECRET FROM LOU'S ARCHIVES

Manufacturers spend much more on the design of the box than they do on the research and development of the products themselves.

SPECIAL VIBRATORS

This list of special vibrators contains brand-name models that have developed quite an avid following across the country.

Hip Harness vibrators. Developed for those who like "hands free" operation of their dildo or vibrator. The main difference between this and the regular handheld vibrators is the design feature of elastic thigh straps, which enable the vibrating area to be adjusted to the lady's liking. This is the same design idea now used for the remote vibrators that a partner can operate across a room. Please be aware that some of these remote vibrators operate on the same radio frequency as garage door openers.

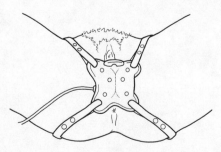

Hip Harness Style

Hitachi Magic Wand. Developed by Hitachi as a body massager, this vibrator has a soft tennis-ball-sized head and gives off strong vibrations. I don't think that Hitachi could have foreseen, in their wildest dreams, their secondary market. This is one of the larger vibrators, and because of its size, women can use it more creatively. For example, a woman can lie facedown on a bed with the wand supported by a couple of pillows under her hips, with the head of the wand strategically placed, while she imagines she is doing her partner.

Pocket Rocket or *Silver Bullet.* These two small vibrators are distinct because of their small size. Let your partner be your guide, as often there is a crucial motion and spot. You may also want to try it on your scrotum, using a soft, circular motion. Or if you prefer a stronger, more direct stimulation, try stroking across the perineal area under the scrotum, aka the taint.

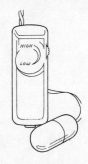

Silver Bullet

Rabbit Pearl. Considered to be the Cadillac of vibrators, the design of the Rabbit Pearl can stimulate both partners at the same time, and you can be in charge of the "remote" control. It has two different operating sections, one vibration and one undulation, which stimulates the vaginal walls. To ensure maximum stimulation for both of you, it's best to concentrate the vibration in the bunny section (leave the

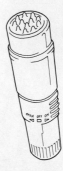

Pocket Rocket

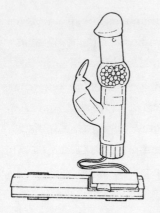

Rabbit Pearl

undulating option off). This way, the lady can have the wand section inserted vaginally and, with you lying on top of her, your hips matched with hers, turn on the (very strong Japanese) motor that operates the bunny section. The RP's nose or ears can be stimulating her clitoral area, and vibration from the back of the Rabbit Pearl can be stimulating the underside of your scrotum.

Micro Clit Tickler. The key to this toy is its stretchy, soft material (same as shaft sleeves). It is designed to be worn by you at the base of your penis so that when you are inside of her, the small, vibrating silver bullet rests over her clitoral area.

G-Spot Vibrator. This vibrator is shaped with an adjustable curving arch so it better reaches the G-spot. Women who love having their G-spot stimulated say they love this style of vibrator.

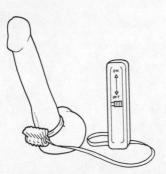

Cyberskin Cock and Clit Tickler

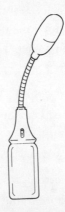

G-Spot Vibrator

Dildos

Dildos, sometimes spelled with an "e" like "potatoes," are typically penis-shaped devices that can do everything a vibrator can except vibrate. And because of their softer texture, dildos have the added benefit of being able to penetrate and provide the sensation of fullness many women love when their partner is busy elsewhere. Dildos are usually made of plastic-like material, rubber, or silicone. They can be made of hard plastic, which is more durable but not as user-friendly and doesn't retain body heat as well.

Like the G-Spot Vibrator, certain dildos have a curved shape to better access a woman's G-spot (through the so-called ceiling, or tummy, side of her vaginal wall). Dildo harnesses are much more popular than you might believe. A harness allows for either partner to be the penetrating or "top" partner. Some men love the novelty of "having my lady strap on some bad leather and do me with a cock harness like I do her"—as a graphic artist from Chicago said. For some couples, the man will wear a harness so he can perform double penetration on his lady. One said, "I can't describe the sensation of my cock inside her and the other 'cock' up her butt. It was mind-blowing. And she gets off on feeling so filled."

One particular toy that utilizes a dildo harness quite efficiently is the Accommodator™, which is essentially a dildo that protrudes from your chin. I know, it looks very unusual, but believe me, your lover may thank you forever. The Accommodator™ is based on the requirement of certain ladies for a form of penetration in order to orgasm during oral sex. As a result, the original design for the Accommodator™ came from eighteenth-century France as an attempt to "improve on nature." In other words, if a man wanted to please a woman using

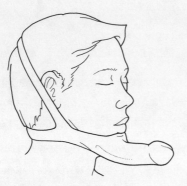

The Accommodator

his tongue, he could also penetrate her with the Accommodator™. This frees up a man's hands and tongue to give his woman pleasure while also "handling" the penetration issue. I admit that when someone tries this on, it is one of the funniest moments of the gentlemen's seminars. You can only imagine the number of times someone shouts "Dickhead!" Yet the men who have actually had the courage to try it said there was no feeling of being restricted or binding from the chin or head straps and that the dildo section stayed in place at the end of their chin . . . just where they wanted it. One man recalled, "When I strap this on, I imagine I am in that French court and only I can do my girl the way she likes." The dildo section measures four inches long with five-inch girth. He can lie down and insert, or she can lower herself onto him when he is in the Sit on My Face (SOMF) position.

Special Play Things

COCK RINGS
(AKA THE CALAMARIS)

Those men who enjoy the sensation of cock rings say it is because of how they build up pressure. Cock rings are based on the law of hydraulics of an erect penis. Stimulation causes blood to flow in and fill the three penis chambers. Gravity and a decrease in stimulation cause the blood to flow back out. Cock rings reduce the drop-off of penile blood pressure by holding shut the veins, along the sides of the erect penis, that allow the blood to flow out. When worn around the penis and under the scrotum, cock rings hold the scrotum away from the body, thereby slowing down ejaculation. These effects combine to result in a firmer, more long-lasting erection, and some men report delays in ejaculation. Those recommended in the men's seminars are made of soft, flexible material, not hard metal.

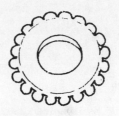

Calamari

HOW TO USE COCK RINGS

1. To be most effective, you or your partner can apply a light lubricant on the ring and your penis. It's best to use a water-based lubricant, as it will not break down the material the way oils/lotions will.

2. The most effective position for the ring is on the shaft and underneath the scrotum. Placing it only on the shaft has some men reporting, "It was too tight just on the shaft, and yet even though I thought the other way would be more of the same, oddly I felt more supported and 'just right.'" It's best that the gentleman does the final adjusting over the testicles.

3. The ring can be worn during manual stimulation by either partner and/or during intercourse. Often couples will try the ring first during manual sex, and when they know what works for them, they move to intercourse.

4. Some couples have reported they enjoyed either starting intercourse with a cock ring on and then removing it prior to climax or placing it on halfway through and finishing with it in place.

5. The scrotum and penis may be a much darker color when the ring is in place. That is natural, as the blood is pooled there. The ring should not be worn for longer than twenty to thirty minutes without removing for a few minutes' break.
6. When you're finished using the cock ring, simply wash with antibacterial soap and water and it will be ready for next time.

SECRET FROM LOU'S ARCHIVES

The cock rings preferred by the field researchers are a soft, flexible material, capable of stretching up to seven inches around.

SHAFT SLEEVES
(AKA THE RIGATONIS)

These one-size-fits-all products are made of a very stretchy, soft, almost plush, rubberlike material that can be used on the penis or fingers. The main idea behind them is that most manual stimulation is done with the fingertips, and those tend to be soft and smooth. Shaft sleeves offer a new way to increase sensation in those most delicate areas with a variety of soft-textured surfaces that are easily controlled with your fingers. Because of their expandable nature, they can also be worn at the base of the penis. In the seminars, men try them on in the palm of their hands and are always surprised by the softness of the sleeves. This versatile item can be used by the:

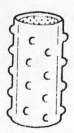

Rigatoni

1. Man on his partner—a boon to men. Now instead of relying solely on your fingertips to stimulate your partner's clitoral area, you have help in the form of these soft-textured sleeves. Just try one on the palm of your hand. Be sure to put the lubricant on or you won't get the real sensation. Men have reported using two at a time so they can caress and pleasure both sides of the inner labia and clitoral ridge. Women say, "He was good with his hands before, and now he is amazing." When used during intercourse, they are worn at the base of the penis for deep, slow penetration. The soft ripples and ridges are able to stimulate the lady. Works for both female-superior and male-superior positions.

2. Woman on her partner—slipped like a finger sleeve over one or two fingertips. Some people report using two sleeves covering different fingers. Apply a light amount of water-based lubricant and use your imagination.

3. Solo—perhaps the best way to discover the sensations possible with the different textures.

SPORTSHEETS™

Like all great ideas, this one began small and then grew. Sportsheets were invented by a marine officer whose inspiration was watching David Letterman attach himself to a wall of Velcro. He said to his officer buddies in the mess, "Wouldn't it be great if you could do that with your girlfriend?" The wife of one of the officers made sheets out of fabric and created Velcro attachment pads with cuffs, and then they had a party to see if this would work. His comment was, "We laughed our asses off," and Sportsheets™ were born.

Sportsheets™ are a kind of sex kit, made up of a very soft, plush, yet durable velour-type sheet that fits a full up to a king-size bed.

Four anchor pads that are attached to cuff straps anchor you or her to the sheet and the bed. The idea is that a woman (or a man) is secured to the bed with the cuffs in whatever position one desires. Of course, you can increase the playfulness of sex without the more serious tone of other dominance and bondage (D&M) products. I call this move the Boy Scout introduction to D&M, for women and men who want to test the waters of bondage in safety.

The fitted sheet is very soft and can be left in place on your bed. The Velcro pads are not at all menacing. For women who like to be "grounded," this is the next best thing to being tied up!

SECRET FROM LOU'S ARCHIVES

For the true bondage beginner, try using toilet tissue to give the feeling of being held hostage, with no real threat.

THE BUNGEE WEIGHTLESS
SEX EXPERIENCE

While this product does not come cheap at $300, it may provide you and yours with a truly new experience . . . just like the name says. Designed by a bungee enthusiast, it is essentially a modified bungee jumping harness, made up of a series of straps that you hang from a stud beam in the ceiling. A photo reference chart for the myriad positions is included in the package.

With her cradled in the harness, you can penetrate her with no back or leg strain. Women and men like the weightlessness. This is the perfect addition to your playground—especially for those of you who like hammocks and swings. There's something about the movement aspect that is exciting and pleasurable. As the designer/inventor said, "Never again will you have a crick in your neck." (Be careful of your drywall. It's best to check before anchoring or you'll tear part of your ceiling out.)

This is also a great way to give her oral sex. With a flick of your finger, you can move her around and never have to crane your neck or move your head again.

LICK-A-LOT-A-PUSS

The package on this product spells out its purpose pretty clearly (as if its title alone didn't do that for you): a "product for the hungry cunnilingus connoisseur." This "labia spreader" is made of soft black leather straps that you fasten around the upper thigh. Each side has a little leather "hand" (the designer's sense of humor showing through) that holds the edge of the outer labia open. The lady can control the degree of openness merely by opening and closing her thighs.

There are three ideas behind this toy. First, spreading the outer labia often results in increased sensation, as the vulvar skin surface is more taut and more available. Second, it avoids the tiredness that both men and women complain of in keeping the labia held open. As one woman said of trying to hold herself open, "I try but I get so slip-

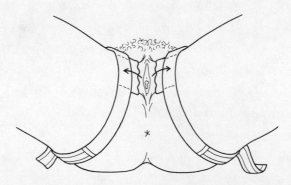

Lick a Lot of Puss

pery I end up digging my nails into my inner lips and that hurts."
Finally, it allows you to free up your hands to do other things.

For those of you who are familiar with a dildo harness, this toy is similar but there is no ring for a dildo. Again, this allows a man's hands to be free to be more creative. The product comes in three colors—black, pink, and purple.

BUTT PLUGS AND ANAL BEADS

For those ladies who enjoy anal stimulation, these are the two favorites. The sensation delivered for women is feeling more full, and if intercourse is to take place, there is an even greater feeling of fullness. For men, the primary stimulation spot is the prostate gland. Both toys require lots of lubrication, as the anal area is nonlubricating.

Butt plugs are in essence a dildo for the anus but with a design adaptation of a flange at the base to ensure it does not fully enter the

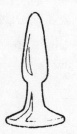

Butt Plug

rectum. It is usually an inverted cone shape so that once it is in, the strength of the sphincter holds it in place. (There are actually two anal sphincters. Only one of the sphincters, the strong muscle ring that keeps the anal opening closed, is under voluntary control. The other is under involuntary control, so try as you might, you can't consciously relax it. Therefore, in order to relax both sphincters, you need physical assistance. One man suggests "inserting one finger for one minute, two fingers for two minutes." But remember to keep the fingers still—don't move them.)

Anal beads are plastic or metal balls on a string. All but one of the beads are inserted into the anus, then pulled out before or at the moment of orgasm, as the PC muscle is undergoing orgasmic spasms in the anus. "When it gets pulled out, I have another orgasmic wave," reported a thirty-seven-year-old woman from Beverly Hills.

Cardinal Toy Rules

1. You need to keep your toys clean. Wash in warm water and an antibacterial soap before and after you use them.
2. Use only water-based lubricants with any of your plastic-compound items, as oil products, massage oil, and hand lotion, for example, will start to break down the surface.
3. Use a condom on parts that are inserted. This makes cleanup a lot easier.
4. Keep toys used for different areas, vaginal/anal, separate from one another. If your lady likes anal penetration, don't use that dildo for her vagina, and so on.
5. Keep your toys in a safe place, away from dust and oils. Toy-savvy types have one bag for vaginal toys and another for anal.
6. Don't share your toys; this is the one time when it is perfectly okay not to share.

Your Toy Chest

Toys can be a wonderful way to add a tone of playfulness and fun to your relationship. By introducing them carefully and gently, you and your partner may discover a new way to please and enjoy one another.

For those of you concerned about your privacy, try storing your toys in a satin pillowcase and slipping it between your mattress and box spring. Use the suggestions in this chapter as a starting point, and know that inventions are being made every day. Enjoy!

Resources
(Where You Can Get the Toys)

In collecting the best sources for toy products, I asked store owners several questions in order to verify their commitment to high quality and an open, encouraging attitude: Did they have a positive sex attitude? Would a woman be comfortable going into the store by herself or ordering over the phone? How big was its selection? Did they sell their mailing list? Was their e-mail site secure?

Catalogs are a great, safe way to introduce tools into the relationship. The very act of choosing a toy can be a bonding, intimate experience. It's a gentle way to suggest what you'd like to try. By looking at the pictures together, you and your partner can feel each other out about what may seem like fun, what may seem too risky, and so on. Initially, making suggestions can make you and her feel vulnerable. Women especially fear being rejected. Remember, gentlemen, they don't want to risk being perceived as "loose," if they suggest using a sex toy.

Essentially, the catalogs I am recommending are tasteful. A couple of these outfits are more oriented toward women, provide wonderful support staff to answer questions via an 800 number, and have careful explanations in the catalogs themselves. Other catalogs are a bit more edgy and less pristine.

WEST COAST

Seattle

Toys in Babeland
707 Pike St., Seattle WA 98122
206-328-2914
Catalog: 800-658-9119
E-mail: *biglove@babeland.com*
Web site: *babeland.com*

> This is a female-run store, originally created as a place for women
> and their comfort. It now carries some male-oriented products.

San Francisco

Good Vibrations
Retail stores:
1210 Valencia St., San Francisco CA 94110
2502 San Pablo Ave., Berkeley CA 94702
Mail order:
938 Howard St., Suite 101, San Francisco CA 94103
415-974-8990
800-289-8423 (in the U.S.)
Fax: 415-974-8989
E-mail: *goodvibe@well.com*
Web site: *http://www.goodvibes.com*

> Good Vibrations is one of the best all-around store/catalog
> combinations. Their specialty is vibrators—and they have an
> endless supply and selection. They also offer a vast array of lu-
> bricants, special massage oils, and videos and books. The se-

lection of toys and leather goods is also of high quality, durability, and inventive styling. All their products have passed customer satisfaction tests. The staff is known for its courteous, nonjudgmental, sex-positive attitude, offering sensitive, knowledgeable, and helpful service.

Los Angeles

The Pleasure Chest
7733 Santa Monica Blvd., Los Angeles CA 90046
323-650-1022
Order line: 800-753-4536
Fax: 323-650-1176
Web site: *www.thepleasurechest.com*

This Pleasure Chest targets a primarily gay male clientele, with a strong leather focus, though straight men and women may find some interesting, curious toys here.

Condomania
7306 Melrose, Los Angeles CA 90046
323-933-7865
Order line: 800-9CONDOMS (U.S. only)
323-930-5330 (for ordering outside the U.S.)
Fax: 323-934-9784
Web site: *www.condomania.com*

This phone/male-order service is one of the best sources for ordering condoms by mail. They offer a selection of over three hundred different condoms. The e-mail site is secure.

Glow

8358 ½ West 3rd St., Los Angeles CA 90048

323-782-9080

E-mail: *glowspotLA@aol.com*

Glow offers an outstanding selection of aromatherapy products.

The Love Boutique

18637 Ventura Blvd., Tarzana CA 91356

818-342-2400

2924 Wilshire Blvd., Santa Monica CA 90403

310-453-3459

Toll-free ordering: 888-568-4663

The two stores are female owned and operated and are open seven days a week. While they offer a small selection of items, the customer is treated with care by a knowledgeable staff. The staff seems uniquely focused on making women feel more at ease and comfortable with their sexuality.

San Diego

F Street Stores (ten stores in the San Diego area)

751 Fourth Ave., San Diego CA 92101

619-236-0841

2004 University Ave., San Diego CA 92104

619-298-2644

7998 Miramar Rd., San Diego CA 92126

619-549-8014

1141 Third Ave., Chula Vista CA 92011

619-585-3314

237 East Grand, Escondido CA 92023

619-480-6031

The stores in this chain offer a wide range of male and female products; it was also one of the first to creat a women's novelty section.

Condoms Plus

1220 University Ave., San Diego CA 92103

619-291-7400

This is a store "with a woman in mind." It is a general license store for all sorts of gifts, as well as condoms. In other words, you can buy a stuffed animal for your child as well as an adult novelty item for your husband. The novelties, however, are in their own section of the store.

MIDWEST

Chicago

The Pleasure Chest (affiliated with the store in New York)

3155 North Broadway, Chicago IL 60657

773-525-7152

Catalog sales: 800-316-9222

The majority of customers are women and couples. This is the store that defined what an adult store should be like: clean, bright, tastefully presented, with nonjudgmental salespeople who look like you and me. This and the New York store (see below) show the impact of being run and operated by the owner, who focuses on taking good care of the customer.

Erotic Warehouse
1246 West Randolph, Chicago IL 60607
312-226-5222

> The store's motto is "We never, ever close." Housed in the warehouse section of town (down the street from Harpo productions), this store has video booths in the back for its customers.

Frenchy's
872 North State St., Chicago IL 60611
312-337-9190

> This store has just undergone a major renovation in appearance and size. It is now three times larger and offers a range of products for men and women.

Minneapolis/St. Paul

Fantasy House Gifts
716 West Lake Street, Minneapolis MN 55408
612-824-2459
Web site: *www.fantasygifts.com*

> There are eight Fantasy House stores in the area, including Bloomington, Bernsville, St. Louis Park, Crystal, Fridley, Coon Rapids, and St. Paul—and two stores in New Jersey, Marlton and Turnersville. Adult material and novelties presented with a comfortable Midwestern environment and attitude. They recently added the Condom Kingdom store in Minneapolis to their operation.

Oklahoma

Christies Toy Box
1184 North MacArthur Blvd., Oklahoma City OK 73127
405-942-4622

> Christies is part of a chain of adult stores, ranked number one in
> the state of Oklahoma; stores also exist in Texas.

EAST COAST

New York

The Pleasure Chest
156 Seventh Ave. South (between Charles and Perry),
New York NY 10014
212-242-4185
New York store customer service: 800-643-1025
Catalog sales: 800-316-9222
E-mail: *apleasurechest.com*
Web site: *apleasurechest.com*

> The New York store and its Chicago sister store are both popular,
> classy, and well stocked, with a range of products for both men
> and women, straight and gay.

Eve's Garden
119 West 57th St., Suite 420, New York NY 10019
212-757-8651
Orders: 800-848-3837
Web site: *www.evesgarden.com*

This is a female-owned and -operated store. What the Pleasure Chest did in 1972 for gay male consumers Eve's Garden did for women in 1974. Located in the heart of midtown Manhattan, Eve's Garden is in the least likely of areas. It is known far and wide as the matriarch of feminine-focused, sex-positive merchandising.

Condomania—New York
351 Bleecker St., New York NY 10014
212-691-9442
U.S. national order line: 800-9CONDOM
323-930-5330 (for ordering outside the U.S.)
Fax: 323-934-9784
Web site: *www.condomania.com*
    Nationally, probably the best source for ordering condoms by mail, phone, or e-mail (their e-mail site is secure.) The store itself is friendly and filled with useful novelty items.

Toys in Babeland
94 Rivington St., New York NY 10002
212-375-1701
E-mail: *comments@babeland.com*
Web site: *www.babeland.com*

Any of the listed products in the book can be purchased through The Sexuality Seminars/FRANKLY SPEAKING, INC. All transactions are confidential and we do not sell our mailing list. To purchase products, inquire about Lou Paget's seminar schedule, book a seminar, be placed on the FRANKLY SPEAKING mailing list, or to get more information, call 1-877-SexSeminars (1-877-739-7364).

Purchases can be made by Visa/MasterCard, cash, or check. FRANKLY SPEAKING, INC. shows on all bank statements and is the name under which all correspondence is sent. All product is discreetly packaged and shipped Priority Post unless otherwise requested. The Speciality Sophist-Kits™ gift boxes can arrive in presentation style (open) or closed—for a bigger surprise. They are delivered UPS or Federal Express and are shipped through Artfull Baskets.

For more information, we can reached at:
FRANKLY SPEAKING, INC.
11601 Wilshire Blvd., Suite 500, Los Angeles CA 90025
310-556-3623
E-mail: *LouPaget@aol.com*
Web site: *LouPaget.com*

THE SOUTH

North Carolina

Adam & Eve
PO Box 800, North Carrboro NC 27510
800-765-ADAM (2326)
Customer service: 919-644-1212

This is the biggest mail-order adult products company in the United States. It offers a full range of products.

CANADA

Toronto

Seduction
577 Yonge St., Toronto, ON M4Y 1Z2
416-966-6969

> This recently opened retail operation is the largest adult novelty store in North America, measuring 15,000 square feet on three floors. The customers are well taken care of by young, fresh-faced college women who know what they are selling.

Love Craft
63 Yorkville Ave., Toronto, ON M5R 1B7
416-923-7331
Web site: *www.lovecraftsexshop.com*

Vancouver

Love Nest
161 East 1st St., North Vancouver, BC V7L 1B2
604-987-1175
Web site: *lovenest.ca*

> As we are going to press, Tony and Kira, the husband/wife owner-operators, were just opening their second store in Whistler, BC.

Calgary

The Love Boutique
9737 MacLeod Trail S., Calgary, AB T2J 0P6
403-252-1846

Just For Lovers
Store #1
920 36th St. NE, #114
403-273-6242
Store #2
4014 MacLeod Trail S.
403-243-2554
Store #3
1415 17th Ave. SW
403-245-9505
Store #4
3630 Brentwood Rd. NW, #515
403-282-7125

·

EIGHT

Capturing Miss O

The Magical Orgasm

This chapter is about the Big O and its potential magic. Specifically, it's about *her* orgasm and what you, as her expert lover, need to take into consideration in order to bring her to orgasm, increase the depth of her sensation, and discover new ways that she can come. Although my main focus is on her, I have also addressed your orgasm, providing you with ways you may enhance your longevity or learn how to better control your timing—two issues men in my seminars have voiced concern about.

Orgasms can be wonderful, transporting, exhausting, and relieving. And for both sexes they can also come too quickly, take forever, feel elusive, and not occur at all. Orgasms are the most natural thing in the world and yet are one of the most anxiety-provoking when they don't happen as easily as we think they should. When it comes to orgasms, we are often held hostage to unnecessary and often debilitating pressure:

➤ To perform
➤ To orgasm multiplely

- To come in the right sequence
- To come the way others do
- To come together

In particular, many women feel pressure to respond. "My old boyfriend was always so concerned that I 'came' that I started faking. I felt so pressured, I couldn't enjoy myself. He felt he had to give me 'one,' and whenever we headed for the bedroom, I began to feel performance anxiety. He didn't believe me when I said I was fine not coming. His need for me to come broke us up." Just take a look at a woman's magazine, where there are endless articles asking women to evaluate themselves with questions such as, "Do you consider yourself highly orgasmic or regularly orgasmic? For clitoral, vaginal, or G-spot orgasms?" As one woman put it, "Good God, how would I know? All I know is what happens with me—not what everyone else is having happen."

In a recent study published in the *New York Times*, when asked whether they had ever experienced orgasm during any kind of sexual activity, whether oral, manual stimulation, or intercourse, 26 percent of women said they regularly did not have orgasms, 23 percent of women said sex was not pleasurable, and 33 percent of men said they had persistent problems climaxing early.

What do these statistics mean? First, they show the high level of sexual dissatisfaction in American men and women. Second, they are an indirect reflection of how much pressure many men and women feel to have orgasms. Indeed, a recent study in *JAMA* (The Journal of the American Medical Association, August 1999) stated that sexual dysfunction is "highly associated with negative experiences in sexual relationships and overall well-being." Both studies confirm and reinforce the psychological and emotional dimension of sexuality, which is especially true of women. Specifically, there is a direct correlation between how nervous or uptight she feels and how easily or controllable an orgasm is. However, by looking at how women orgasm, from both a biologic perspective and an emotional one, you will greatly increase your ability to help her to a satisfying, even thrilling, orgasm.

You do her and yourself a disservice by placing so much importance on the act itself, taking away the fun, the pleasure, and the potential thrill. In this way, I agree with Dr. Beverly Whipple, professor at Rutgers University, president of AASECT, and secretary of the World Association of Sexology, who says that whatever we do in this arena should be "a pleasure-oriented sexual experience, not a goal-oriented experience." She also believes, and I agree, that no one has the right to tell another that his or her sexual experiences aren't valid or adequate. We all deserve to experience our own particular orgasms—however and whenever they occur.

A New Approach

So how can we approach the almighty orgasm, take away its mythic proportions, and bring it down to its natural size and place? First, you have to become aware of the feeling of pressure and then commit to reducing it. I think the best way to do this is to take a less goal-oriented approach to making love. The direct result will be that the Big O will lose some of its power. Then—surprise! Often it happens in an even more intense way! A less goal-oriented approach means being open and spontaneous and resisting the focus on or expectation of orgasm. A man, a real estate developer from Houston, pointed to his frustration about too much emphasis on orgasm in this way: "With little kids running around our house, it seems like we never have enough time to take our time. We have to resort to 'mercy fucks' when one of us needs something now. But when we have our Saturday night or Sunday morning sex and can play, it is so different, the feel, the connection, and the orgasms."

Again, if you have already helped your partner relax, in her mind and body, then she is in a much better place to experience an orgasm. A woman lawyer from Pittsburgh told this story: "I had never had an orgasm with a man until my boyfriend at the time, who was this sweet, younger man, went down on me. While he was 'down there,' I thought, 'Well, nothing is going to happen.' Then he said, 'I just want to do this—I love eating you.' So I figured, well, let him go ahead if he's enjoying himself. Ten minutes later—*boom!* Out of left field I had my first orgasm. Now I realize it was because I had just totally relaxed and not been tied to what was supposed to happen. I knew the feel from my hand and vibrator but it was like I needed that to get the nerve pathways opened up to know what to feel and expect. After that I had them regularly from oral sex."

Another woman related this experience: "My lover and I were spending a stolen afternoon together and I just sort of drifted mentally as he played with me clitorally. It was a lazy, quiet day and I was so relaxed by what he was doing, and all of a sudden, the orgasm snuck up on me. It was the first time I'd ever had one honestly with a man." In both cases, these women let go of any expectation or plan and were pleasantly surprised by their orgasms.

Another key that will enable you to help her orgasm is to remember how and why foreplay is so essential to women. As I've mentioned earlier in the book, most women orgasm through manual and oral stimulation. Men generally prefer to "wait" until intercourse to come.

If you approach the whole idea of foreplay as a vital component of sex, not a mere stage before sex (i.e., intercourse), then you may feel more engaged in getting her to where she wants to go instead of focusing on where you're wanting to go next. A bartender from New York said, "Yeah, I love it when she comes, like no kidding, I'm a guy, I love results. But the even bigger turn-on for me is getting her there and knowing I can make my wife feel *that* good. It is the ride that does it for me, not just the finish line." Again, since most men orgasm before women (we will get to the subject of simultaneous orgasm a bit later in the chapter), it's up to you to concentrate on her first. In other words, though she of course wants you to come, you may need to put her before you. If you incorporate this more altruistic attitude into your whole approach to sex, I guarantee you, a woman will return the favor in triplicate.

SECRET FROM LOU'S ARCHIVES

According to noted sex therapists and authors Dr. Michael Riskin and Anita Baker-Riskin, most men orgasm in the first three minutes of intercourse, but can learn to control their climax for up to seven minutes. A woman, if she's going to orgasm, typically takes more time to come. However, some women can orgasm within three to seven minutes of stimulation.

Getting her to that place of no return is 95 percent determination and dedication and 5 percent talent. The talent portion is very straightforward and simply requires that you know the topography of the area and your partner's likes and dislikes.

Timing

As I said above, since most women can or are used to orgasming through oral or manual stimulation, they tend to come before men. This is not a rule, it's merely a standard operating procedure that most men and women use when it comes to sex. However, you may want to consider shaking up this sex formula by asking, "Who wants to go first?" You may be pleasantly surprised by what you discover. For example, a number of women in my seminars put off coming until they are penetrated. An architect from Dallas said, "The more aroused I get, the more I want him inside of me." Another seminar attendee stated, "There are times when I absolutely crave having him inside of me. I may have already had an orgasm from being eaten, but I don't feel complete until he's inside me." Another woman said it more succinctly. "Oh God, sometimes I just grab him and say, 'Now, I want you in me now!'" My point here is twofold. First, although the exact trigger for the orgasm may be your fingers or your lips on her, the feeling or experience of the orgasm *extends* beyond that time. Second, for many women it's your penetration of her that *completes* the feeling of the orgasm.

Another aspect of timing that you might want to keep in mind is the very consistent biological fact that women cycle. Sometimes her cycle asserts itself as a wonderful feat of nature, making her want you unexpectedly and intensely. Other times you may want to curse Mother Nature, as your partner seems distant, irritable, or just plain uninterested in sex. By now, I'm sure you all have heard of PMS (premenstrual syndrome), during which some women suffer drastic mood swings, while others experience no real symptoms. But, gentlemen, you need to understand that these swings of temperament (and sexual readiness) are very much part of her biology. Now, sometimes not being in the mood may be about being tired and grumpy, but sometimes it may have an even realer relationship to where she is in her cycle.

The obvious sign of a woman's cycle is her monthly menses, or period. Between puberty and menopause, healthy women menstruate on a cyclic basis, every twenty-four to thirty-two days. Although most people are aware only of the days of a woman's menstrual flow (her period), these days are only the most obvious stage in the complete reproductive cycle. A cycle begins on the first day of a menstrual cycle and ends when the next cycle's flow starts. Essentially, the first phase of a woman's cycle, called the follicular phase, lasts up to twelve days, beginning with the first day of her period. During this time she sheds the lining of her uterus, causing bleeding. Most women bleed for three to five days and some experience cramping— in differing degrees. This is usually a good time for sex for two reasons: (1) If she has an orgasm, she may alleviate some cramping of the uterus, and (2) there is a very reduced chance of her getting pregnant. At the end of this phase, endorphins peak and increased estrogen gives her ample vaginal lubrication. In the morning her endorphins are highest.

Some women and men experience uneasiness about having sex while a woman is bleeding. In some cases, this reluctance is related to a taboo that goes back at least to the Old Testament when a woman's blood was considered "unclean" and it was therefore "bad" to have sex at this time. Even today, many women prefer to avoid having sex during their period because they find it messy or uncomfortable. Women also worry that men will be turned off by the sight, feel, or smell of blood. Some of the messiness is unavoidable, as condoms and blood, in particular, don't mix well, creating vaginal dryness and possibly causing a tear in the condom. A possible solution is to use Instead, a vaginal cup that acts as a diaphragm.

Men have also voiced their worries about it being "all right" or safe to have sex at this time. My advice to you, gentlemen, is this: If you don't mind, you should encourage her to be open and receptive about sex. You may want to tell her that you don't mind her bleeding. Such an attitude can be a wonderful feeling of acceptance. One sports marketing executive said, "I don't care. It's my wife who thinks it's awful. I like her body all the time. I am her man twenty-eight days a month."

The next phase is the ovulatory phase, which lasts for three days, between days 13 and 15. This is when she's in full baby-making mode. An indicator for most women is seeing the egg-white-like mucus in their secretions. An egg moves into one (or two) of her fallopian tubes, and her cervical mucus thins, making it easier for sperm to reach the egg. Some experts say women produce more testosterone in this phase, creating a stronger sex drive in these three days.

The luteal phase takes place in days 16 to 30. If she gets pregnant in the ovulatory phase, this is the time for the fertilized egg to respond and grow. She produces progesterone, a hormone that thickens the uterine lining and inhibits endorphins that would throw off proper fertilization. As you may be familiar, at this time of the month she may feel irritable because of the cryptic yet real PMS, which usually ends with the onflow of bleeding.

Now, gentlemen, when it comes to your timing and how it affects her, I have heard, again and again, cries of frustration. Most of you first learn to orgasm by masturbating, which, of course, is perfectly natural. However, because masturbation is all about you, and you know just what to do in order to bring yourself to climax, you tend to come quickly. Consequently, if you're used to coming quickly, then it's hard to break the habit when you're aroused with a woman. The nerve pathways have already been established, and you have to consciously learn how to control your timing. Unfortunately, "quick" has become too often confused with "premature," further offending you guys. In terms of understanding your own timing, things to be considered are premature ejaculation and ways of staying hard. Later in this chapter I will discuss how men can learn to control these timing issues.

SECRET FROM LOU'S ARCHIVES

The definition of premature ejaculation is when a man ejaculates before he wants to.

Types of Female Orgasms

In general, most women experience an orgasm in three areas: the clitoris, vagina, and G-spot. But an orgasm can originate anywhere from the clitoris to the nipples—sometimes even a head massage can create an orgasm. Women are so connected to their minds that with the proper arousal techniques, anything may then stimulate the area of orgasm.

CLITORAL ORGASM

The clitoral orgasm is the number one spot for the most common and often the strongest orgasms in women. Indeed, the majority of women need some form of clitoral stimulation to orgasm. This kind of stimulation can occur manually, orally, with a dildo or vibrator, or during intercourse (see below under "Coital Alignment Technique"). Some women like light, soft touches to become aroused, followed by more intense or fast pressure. Other women prefer to be touched only with soft or only with hard pressure. As always, ask her what she likes or watch her touch herself.

Keep in mind that the majority of women come through manual or oral stimulation of the clitoris, not penetration. If a woman prefers vaginal penetration while being stimulated clitorally, the female-superior position provides the most direct control. (See Chapter Nine for more information regarding positions.)

SECRET FROM LOU'S ARCHIVES

The clitoris is the only feature of the human body whose function is solely for pleasure.

G-SPOT ORGASM

I'm assuming, gentlemen, that you remember the guide I provided you earlier and can now locate her G-spot. For those of you who need a quick refresher, Dr. Beverly Whipple, the woman who coined the term "G-spot," says you can find this delicious spot by imagining the inside of her vagina as a small clock, with twelve o'clock pointing toward the navel. The G-spot is generally located between eleven and one o'clock. Unlike the clitoris, which protrudes from its hood, the G-spot lies above the vaginal walls surrounding the urethra and is barely noticeable unless a woman is aroused. Dr. Whipple says that one of the most misunderstood facts about the G-spot is that it is not *in* the vaginal wall, but rather can be felt *through* the vaginal wall, along the course of the urethra. A second misconception is that the G-spot is almost always associated with women ejaculating.

You can help her locate her G-spot by inserting your finger gently into her vagina and curving it up toward the tummy. She can also do this herself in a squat position, and remember that some form of arousal is necessary to feel it. But as Dr. Bernie Zilbergeld, the author of *New Male Sexuality*, told me, "There is no need to be held hostage by having to find it."

Try using your finger in a "come here" motion, with a specifically shaped dildo/vibrator, or during penetration. The best positions for G-spot stimulation during intercourse are:

1. Rear entry
2. Woman superior—either facing toward the man or, often better, facing his feet
3. Male superior—with the woman putting her legs over her partner's arms or shoulders. In this position a man with a prow-shaped penis actually has a better chance of stimulating the G-spot because of his curvature. Some men with straighter erections use a strong arching-back position to attain that same angle.

SECRET FROM LOU'S ARCHIVES

Some researchers report that nearly 40 percent of women had experienced at least one ejaculation at orgasm, while others found a much smaller percentage. (*The Kinsey Institute New Report on Sex*, 1990)

VAGINAL ORGASM

This form of orgasm uses the same nerve pathways as the G-spot, the hypogastric and pelvic. Now that you are aware that the clitoris is much larger than it appears, its legs extending alongside the vaginal walls, you probably understand that women can experience an orgasm vaginally.

This can also occur by contracting the PC muscle during penetration. A rhythmic pulsing motion—either short, quick pulses or longer, slower pulses—can stimulate the nerve endings. Women describe this as a very deep, pushing-out style of orgasm.

COITAL ALIGNMENT TECHNIQUE

Also known as CAT, this technique requires the alignment of two parts of the genitals: her clitoris and the pubic bone region at the base of your penis. The man's pubic area is cushioned by fat tissue, so it isn't just hard bone. If a man is deep enough inside, and maintains constant contact between her clitoris and his pubic bone, a woman can achieve an orgasm when he uses a gentle rocking motion. In this way, he is maintaining contact with her clitoris, with added stimulation of penetration. The typical thrusting in and out of male superior doesn't maintain enough constant contact with the clitoral area to have that be a way for most women to orgasm.

"C" (CERVICAL) ORGASM

For some women a deep and constant pressure on the cervix can lead to orgasm. It would be the pelvic hypogastric nerve pathway that is stimulated with this pressure. Some women who enjoy fisting say they enjoy having the cervix held.

"U" (URETHRAL) ORGASM

Given what we now know about the size and dimension of the clitoris, it makes sense that for some women stimulation of the urethra would be highly pleasurable. After all, it is surrounded on three sides by the clitoral body. Located between the clitoral glans and the vaginal opening (introitus), the urethra is stimulated during the thrusting action of intercourse, as well as during oral and manual stimulation, when one can use more refined and direct motions.

Aside from the so-called usual ways females orgasm, women are also known to come in quite imaginative ways, ranging from touching of the nipples to fantasy, to rubbing their clitoris on their partner's leg,

---

SECRET FROM LOU'S ARCHIVES

The majority of women report orgasming most regularly with oral sex or manual stimulation.

---

to being spanked. (Although I am aware of women who also love bondage and S&M orgasms, I will leave such discussions to those with more expertise in that area.) Here are some not-so-typical orgasms.

BREAST ORGASM

This is not a Ripley's Belive It or Not—I promise. Some women have reported that the licking and manual stimulation of their breasts and nipples can get them so excited that they come. I think it's a testament to the sensitivity of our skin and our minds!

SECRET FROM LOU'S ARCHIVES

"What we do know is that each woman seems to have her own orgasmic pattern. This pattern is so individual that Hartman, Fithian, and Campbell, respected sex therapists and researchers, call this individuality 'orgasmic fingerprinting.' Each woman's orgasmic pattern is as unique as her fingerprints." (Dr. Lonnie Barbach)

ALL-OVER BODY STIMULATION

Some women report that all-over body stimulation can lead to an orgasm. Now, they may feel the actual orgasm in the pelvis, but it is your roving hands, fingers, and tongue that build the sensation.

FEMALE EJACULATION

Some women when they orgasm or experience a deep orgasm will also feel a gush of fluid. This is not urine. This is an expression of fluid from the paraurethral glands. There are approximately 150 Skene's glands ducts (also called paraurethral glands) that lead into the urethra—"para" meaning that these glands are on the sides of the urethra. In studies performed by Dr. Paco Cabello, a Spanish researcher, urine samples were collected from women before and after stimulation without a male partner, and he found that there was PSA—prostate specific antigen—in the urine post-stimulation. This is another reason to refer to the G-spot area as the female prostate.

Some women ejaculate regularly, some occasionally, and some never, although according to research by Dr. Cabello, because the amount of ejaculant is so small (2 to 3 ccs), it might just be considered normal vaginal secretions and therefore not obvious.

SECRET FROM LOU'S ARCHIVES

Both men and women have love muscles, the PC muscles that, if toned, can enhance orgasm. And like any muscle, these can be exercised, and one need not go to the gym. When a man tightens his PC muscle, his penis will jump up and down. A woman can tighten her PC muscles by stopping the flow of urine. A good male exercise is placing a washcloth on your erect penis and doing penis lift-ups.

One man from my seminar recalled how when he began stimulating his partner's nipples, she became "phenomenally wet." "She just started flowing, soaking through not only the sheets but the mattress pad as well," he explained, "and then when I went down on her, there was this squishing sound—made more obvious because there wasn't all that much to listen to down there." This story goes to show you that some women respond to the slightest touch.

It's on the Chromosome

I feel it's necessary to say yet again that men and women are different, and this difference is very clear in the arena of the orgasm. Both men and women have two separate nerve pathways for orgasms, the pudendal and the pelvic. It is because there are these two pathways that men and women can experience climax differently.

Specifically, as Dr. Lonnie Barbach says in her book *For Each Other*, "The pudendal nerve supplies the clitoris, PC muscle, inner lips, skin of the perineum, and skin surrounding the anus. The pelvic nerve goes to the vagina and the uterus. The fact that the pudendal nerve has considerably more sensory fibers than the pelvic nerve and contains the kind of nerve endings which are very sensitive to touch may be responsible for the higher percentage of women being more responsive to clitoral stimulation. The two-nerve theory may account for more than differences between vaginally induced and clitorally induced orgasms. Because these two nerves partially overlap in the spinal cord, it may also account for blended orgasms which are both clitorally and vaginally induced."

In women, clitoral orgasms go along the pudendal nerve pathway;

vaginal and G-spot orgasms go along the pelvic nerve pathway. With clitoral orgasms there is a pulling-up sensation, and with vaginal and G-spot there is a pushing-down sensation. For men, the stimulation of the penis is along the pudendal pathway, and the male G-spot/prostate stimulation is along the pelvic pathway. Now, isn't it nice to get that straightened out?

SECRET FROM LOU'S ARCHIVES

Blended orgasms are when both sexual nerve pathways are stimulated at the same time: for women the clitoris and the G-spot, and for men the penis and the prostate.

Male Orgasm

Don't worry, I didn't forget you. It's simply that I understand that in this department you are probably very familiar with how to accomplish your own orgasm. However, I would like to address certain issues and techniques that may be of interest in terms of learning how better to maintain your erection and give her more pleasure.

In essence, a man's orgasm has two parts to it. According to Dr. Barbara Keesling in her book *How to Make Love All Night*, the first phase is the emission phase, during which the cannon loads with the seminal fluid that has been collected in the prostate. Next is the expulsion phase, during which the cannon fires the ejaculate out of the body, creating rhythmic waves throughout the body. The entire ejaculation process, emission and expulsion, takes about two seconds. As Keesling says, "It is very important for you to have a full understanding of your own ejaculatory process, including the timing, if you are going to be a master of your own body. For most men, the contraction of the PC during expulsion is an involuntary process. Once you take control of your PC muscle, however, you can voluntarily delay or prevent ejaculation." This is a progressive learning process that a man can do by himself or with a partner. The main aim is for a man to exercise his PC muscles (using the washcloth-lift, for example). He will then experience more control during penetration and thrusting. The result is multiorgasmic men and increased sexual stamina and control.

Men seem unnecessarily concerned with how many times a night they can have sex and orgasm. Listen to most women and they will tell you once is enough if it's done right. However, gentlemen, you may be interested in knowing that as men age, the number of times per night typically drops to once. There aren't hard statistics, because there aren't any scientific studies, but these numbers do correspond to my anecdotal information. The norm for most men is one time, and typically as a man ages, his refractory time (the time in between erections) lengthens. However, there are men for whom there is very little change between the refractory time and/or strength of their erections throughout their lives.

SECRET FROM LOU'S ARCHIVES

And so you know, gentlemen, ladies for the most part know you masturbate. What they may not know is *why* you're masturbating. They might think you are not sexually satisfied; they think something is wrong with the love or the sexual relationship and may believe that something is missing. You need to let them know that nothing can replace them.

ENHANCERS

Though many women don't even want you to stay erect for hours (after all, sustained penetration can lead her to soreness and irritation), there are ways you can improve your lasting power.

➤ Cock rings not only can enhance her pleasure, by making you feel more full inside of her, but can increase the intensity of your feeling as well. Be sure to put the cock ring over both the shaft of your penis and the scrotum. Some men like to take it off just as they are about to come; other men prefer leaving the cock ring on. Men claim that the cock ring, which helps build up pressure, increases the sensation during intercourse.

➤ The Squeeze Technique: While you're erect, squeeze your penis right below the head. This will help slow you down, enabling you to prolong sex. You can also have her do this for you.

➤ Desensitizing spray: I don't usually recommend these products, as they have a numbing active ingredient, benzocaine. However, men use these sprays to literally make them last longer when they want to have multiple sessions.

➤ Viagra: This pharmaceutical phenomenon is meant for men who clinically suffer from impotence or penile erectile dysfunction and should only be used under a doctor's supervision. Though the wide reports stress how Viagra is a "miracle" that lets men remain erect for hours, I have also heard reports of its misuse. After taking two Viagra, one young man in his early twenties had three orgasms and still remained erect. Remaining erect for too long can lead to permanent damage of the penile tissue, which is known as priapism.

PENIS ENLARGEMENT TECHNIQUES

There are essentially two techniques that enhance the length or girth of your penis. Again, both techniques come with important caveats.

1. Surgery that cuts the suspensory ligaments at the top of the penis will make the penis look longer when soft. The end result, however, is that when the penis is erect, it loses some of its stability and has been known to "wobble."

2. An injection of adipose (fatty) tissue taken from another area of the man's body into the penis is used to enlarge one's girth. However, it has been known to "look weird." Moreover, the adipose tissue is often reabsorbed irregularly by the body, causing the penis to become "lumpy" and malformed.

- ➤ Some men have full orgasms when soft.
- ➤ Some men love a blended orgasm—the simultaneous stimulation of penis and G-spot/prostate.
- ➤ Some men have dry orgasms, in which they have the full sensation of coming, without releasing any ejaculate. This occurs for one of two reasons: either he controls (i.e., suppresses) ejaculation or, after a tremendous amount of activity, there's "nothing left in the tanks."
- ➤ Men fake orgasms, too. If they think they are not going to come, they have been known to suddenly pull a groin muscle or get a stomachache.

Multiple and Simultaneous Orgasms

Though I don't think the media have intentionally misled us about orgasm, they have reinforced and perpetuated certain inaccuracies. In its hungry quest for information about the heady subject of sex, the media have often rushed to the proverbial table with half-baked goods. So I have two purposes here: first, to debunk some of the myths surrounding sex, specifically about the multiple and the simultaneous orgasm; and second, to encourage you to explore and try new approaches—for if we don't challenge ourselves, how will we ever know what's possible?

The main reason to debunk myths is built into the nature of myths. By its very definition, a myth contains a grain of truth on which an entire beach has been created. There have been so many articles written about the fabulous multiple or simultaneous orgasm. Do they occur? Yes for some and never for others.

In the seminars, those men and women who say they have simultaneous orgasms are invariably in long-term relationships where they are very aware of one another's bodies and sexual responses. A nurse from Lexington, Kentucky, said, "I am Spanish and was raised very Catholic. I was a virgin when I got married and had no understanding or knowledge about sex. Yet with my husband, we can often come together; I thought everyone did. But it wasn't until my American girlfriends told me that [coming together] was uncommon that I realized I was an exception. I now know that the reason it happens for us is we are so tuned to one another's bodies."

There are those people, however, who, no matter how much they try, do not experience simultaneous orgasms. Often this is because of their physiologies. In other words, because of their shape, men may not be able to "hit" her in the right spot, or women can only orgasm through direct clitoral stimulation, which is often difficult during intercourse. So, gentlemen, do not feel inadequate if simultaneous orgasm is not part of your sexual repertoire.

An investment banker from Boston said, "I finally decided to stop keeping up with the Joneses sexually. It was making me and my husband stressed with always trying to do what was in books and make things 'work.' I wanted to try something new, but I went too far. Now it is fun to look and say sure let's try, and if it works, great, and if it doesn't, well that's not for us."

There are ways both men and women can practice or train their bodies to be more responsive or ready for multiple orgasms. Start with exercising your PC muscle and getting it into shape. The PC muscle is slung from the front to the back of the pelvic girdle in both sexes. Men have two holes through it, the anus and the urethra, whereas women have three: the anus, vagina, and urethra. It is the control of the expulsion phase of the man's orgasmic response that enables him to become multiorgasmic. In women, it's a strong PC muscle that enables them to come more powerfully. Women are naturally more capable of being multiorgasmic, in part because their orgasm is not tied to ejaculation, which men in the seminars stated takes an enormous amount of energy from a man.

But it remains true that for most couples, multiple and simultaneous orgasms don't happen often, easily, or without hard work. Please note the operative term—work.

A man's ability to satisfy and share with his partner in many ways is the real test of his lovemaking skill. Creating an orgasm is just one. Therefore, though you may agree that achieving an orgasm does not necessarily equal satisfaction, it is often our immediate and most important barometer or scale that we use to measure whether or not the sex was "good." Some people even claim they really haven't made love if one or both of them don't come. Instead of judging your lovemaking, enjoy it. An orgasm is meant to delight both of you, not be a barometer of your pleasure.

— • —

NINE

Nights of Nirvana: Intercourse That Will Leave Her Breathless

Deep Connection

You've led her to the place of ultimate relaxation and romance; you've moved her to the heights of arousal through oral and manual sex, perhaps even including some fun with toys; now it's time to push her over the top with the most sensual, soulful intercourse imaginable. Ultimately, we all want to get to this place, where deep connection feels complete. I believe a woman's desire is often best fulfilled with you inside of her, leaving her breathless and sated. One woman said, "Sometimes it is almost overwhelming, my wanting to have him inside of me—like now! There is nothing that compares to the feeling of when he first enters me."

In order to be a master lover during intercourse, a few premises must be acknowledged. First, you need to take into consideration your attitude in general. A woman wants to know not only that you find her attractive and want her but that you also respect her. Once this level of comfort and trust is established, then she wants you to take her with abandon.

Second, at this stage, you need to have paid attention to her entire body before you begin to penetrate her. Finally, let go and see what happens. Let your and her body lead you without any preconceived ideas of exactly what will happen.

Most women realize that intercourse is strenuous and requires work and energy. With that in mind, I'd like to share a story with you. A friend of mine and I were hanging out one day discussing sex, and he mentioned how sex can be such hard work for men. When I laughed at this notion, he said, "Okay, Lou, I'm gonna prove something to you, you think I'm kidding." He stood up and walked to the center of the room and plunked down on the rug. He then said, "Okay, I'm the woman, you're the guy, lie on top of me." With a quizzical look on my face, I lay on top of him. He looked up at me and said, "Now, get your hips in the right position; they are not in the right position. Okay, now start thrusting."

I looked down at him and with a look of amazement said, "I didn't know your toes had to be in a certain position in order to push. This hurts the abs."

He nodded and said, "Keep thrusting and be careful not to put all your weight on me."

By now my arms were exhausted.

He said, "Now keep thrusting, maintain your erection, don't put all your weight on me, and then stare into my eyes and tell me you love me!"

Needless to say, while I collapsed, laughing, I got his message!

But for all this hard work, the beauty of sex remains in the fabulous friction created when bodies move together. The main movement of intercourse will always be the thrusting in and out. But there is a decided art to thrusting well. Here are some of the suggestions I've collected from the ladies' seminars.

1. Please start slowly, very slowly, and build the tempo.
2. Mix short strokes with long and deep.
3. Make different moves with your hips—try wiggles and circles. Often a lady has different areas of vaginal entry with specific pressure sensitivities. Your movement can uncover these hot spots.
4. If you take too long, she will dry out. Sometimes women can enjoy sex for forty-five minutes and sometimes we prefer it in five. Even if a lady is totally turned on and fully lubricated in that area, her tissue is extremely delicate, and once exposed to air, as it is during sex, the friction of thrusting can dry it out, particularly when a condom is used. I can assure you, gentlemen, this does not feel good. Consider a couple of solutions: (1) use a lubricant; (2) after some time, ask her if she is comfortable or if you feel smooth enough.
5. Please stay inside. Once you are in there, we really like you to stay there.

6. Ask her to control the show and ask her to get on top—that way you can get an idea of what she likes and duplicate it when it's your turn.

7. While thrusting, stay close to her clitoral area. Banging on top of the clitoris does nothing. The motions that really work are pelvic rocking and slow circular movement. There is a reason why the pelvic grind works—you are stimulating her clitoris.

SECRET FROM LOU'S ARCHIVES

I now know why the ab machines at the gym are so popular and why almost every men's magazine publishes methods for strengthening your back: The stronger your abs, the less likely you are to stop halfway through intercourse, collapsing in exhaustion.

Does Your Size Really Matter?

Well, I won't lie to you. There are some real size queens out there. They may not measure you, but they definitely have their preferences. Some women like very small penises, in part because they have small vaginas. For other women, the larger the penis, the better. Just like men can be "breast" men or "ass" men, women have their share of preferences. But for many women, it's what you do with your penis that really matters.

Most men are smaller erect than you think. Take, for example, the four sizes of instructional product (i.e., dildos) I use in the ladies' sex seminars. When I place them all in the center of the table and instruct the women to choose the size they are most comfortable with, most often they choose the five-inch executive model or the six-inch model because that's the size with which they are most familiar.

That said, it's true that women see your erections from a completely different angle than you do. We see from below, where it is bigger, see? In that way, you could say that we have the home-court advantage. It's all a matter of perception.

SECRET FROM LOU'S ARCHIVES

The smaller he is, the closer in he has to remain, which is a very good thing. And a smaller man can use deep-penetrating positions with a woman because he won't be ramming into her cervix.

Positions

Don't let these "1001 Positions" books overwhelm or distract you or make you feel inadequate because there are some positions you haven't even heard of. Please remember that the biggest determining factor for choosing a position is the preference of you and your partner. Note that most of the positions in porn movies are not at all pleasurable for the ladies. One male friend of mine said he'd watch films in order to gauge his own performance. When I told him that these performances were scripted, acted, voiced-over, and edited, he seemed shocked. And this reaction came from a television producer!

Couples typically use two or three positions during one lovemaking session, moving from one position to another before completion, whether completion is orgasm or not. Nevertheless, I don't want you thinking that there is something wrong with you or your lover because you prefer your old standard of you on top and her beneath you. Above all, do what is comfortable and what works best for both of you in terms of pleasure. While I do encourage variety in all forms of sexual intimacy, the purpose is to push back the boundaries of self-imposed limitations and find your ultimate pleasure.

Essentially, there are only six positions, with everything else being a variation on a theme: man on top, woman on top, side by side, rear entry, standing, and sitting/kneeling.

MAN SUPERIOR (MAN ON TOP)

In the man-superior position, you are on top during intercourse. This is one of the most common positions and one women and men often enjoy the most. This preference is mostly because of the position's degree of closeness and the ability to watch each other's expressions and look into each other's eyes. You're also able to sense and feel your partner better and make her feel most connected to you.

The name of the so-called missionary position is ascribed to South Seas natives who saw the missionaries doing this. The South Seas tribes saw man on top as different because they favored woman on top, sitting, and rear entry. (According to Kinsey, those of us who are of European descent seem to rely on the missionary position as an old standard.)

In this position, the woman lies on her back with the man lying over her or slightly to the side of her. Men say they like it because they can control the depth of penetration as well as the speed of the thrust, according to how close they are to orgasm. Women like the position because there is more body contact than in the other positions. While the other positions are perhaps more erotic, this one is the most romantic. Kissing and hugging are easily done in this position, and many women say it makes them feel safe and protected.

This position is also good for coital alignment technique (CAT). In Position A, observe a variation on the positioning of the feet that can add greatly to coital alignment technique, in which you brace your feet against hers. By keeping your hips together so your pubic area is in continuous contact with her clitoral and vulvar areas, there is no break in the stimulation or connection, and you can penetrate her most deeply. She can assist this by firmly holding your buttocks. Now, this is all fine and good as long as a man can maintain motion, which is difficult because he is not using his knees and feet for leverage. Look at the feet in the drawing. See how her legs are fairly close together (about a foot apart) and she holds her feet out to the sides with her toes toward the outer edges of the bed? As it was explained to me, once she has her feet and legs in this position, a man can use the top of her flexed feet to brace himself. This is perfect for those close, constant pelvic thrusts that make the CAT. It's also desirable for those women who enjoy and need muscular tension to orgasm. If the man is taller, the same can be achieved by using a wall or bed footboard as the brace.

I call the following the BTS (Better Than Sex) variation of Position A, for the more athletic. It allows you to maintain full body contact while increasing pelvis pressure/tension, and allows a greater ability to create tight close-thrusting motions because he is using both legs as a fulcrum. This is how it's done:

Step 1: The man has entered the woman, and then he squeezes her legs together with his on the outside.

Man Superior

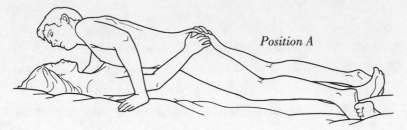

Position A

Position B

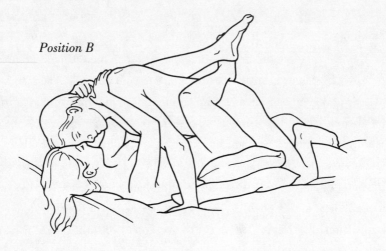

Position C

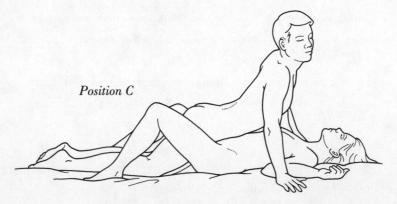

Step 2: He then bends his knees and hooks his ankles underneath the woman's legs.

Step 3: He lifts his legs up, and in doing so gently lifts up her legs, increasing pelvis/clitoral pressure while maintaining full, warm body contact.

In Position B the lady rests against a pillow. Think of this as a perfect sex toy under her hips to increase her vaginal entry angle. The pillow creates a nice and relaxing spot for her back and makes it easier for the man to thrust vigorously and still remain inside. Fewer spills or "fall-outs" occur when pillows are used. With her legs wrapped over his hips, she can also control the motion and open herself to more penetration. Need I mention that this position also allows great access for kissing?

In Position C the man is arching back, which is a great boon for women who enjoy more front-vaginal-wall/G-spot stimulation and stroking, and who aren't comfortable with rear-entry sex. This is not a good position for a man with a bad back, but it does enable the man with tight ab muscles to show off his ripples.

SECRET FROM LOU'S ARCHIVES

Any kind of exercise, including sex, can help abort an impending headache.

WOMAN SUPERIOR (WOMAN ON TOP)

Many women prefer woman superior because it allows her to control penetration and the speed, since she is the person doing the thrusting. It also works well if a woman happens to be taller/smaller than you. In Position A, the woman is doing the same to the gentleman

Woman Superior

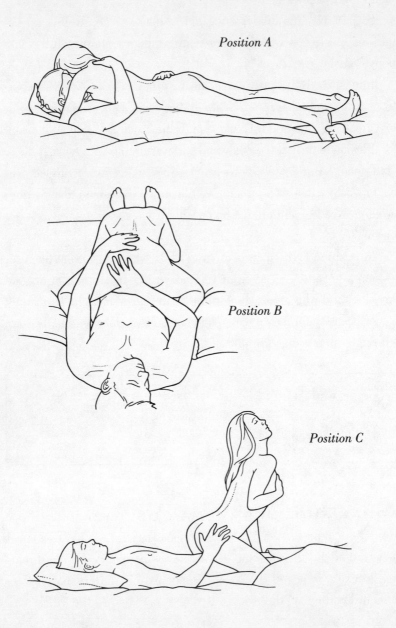

Position A

Position B

Position C

that he was doing to her in man-superior Position A above. She uses his feet to brace herself for close clitoral and pelvic rocking, and because her legs are on the inside, she can create more pressure on the vulvar and clitoral areas by squeezing her legs.

In the woman-superior position, she is usually straddling him with the bulk of her weight distributed evenly between both knees. This can be done with her either facing you or facing away from you (Position C). Another variation on this position would be for her to lie down on you with her legs on either side (Position B). The woman-superior position does require a lot more work on a woman's part, and some say it requires a "ski racer's quads." Men tend to enjoy this position a lot because it provides them with a good look at a woman's body; you can be the captain of the proverbial ship. They love to see a woman's breasts move up and down with each thrust and see her hair falling or hitting them in the chest or face. A magazine editor from San Francisco remembers: "I knew this would be my favorite position from the time I saw a porn film when I was fourteen when this woman in a big skirt lowered herself onto a man. When my wife lowers herself onto me, it takes all my power not to shoot off right then."

In general, women find the variations of this position exciting because they allow them to control movement and the depth of penetration. They feel like they are running the show, so to speak. On the other hand, the women who don't enjoy this position say that it's because they feel self-conscious about having their bodies exposed and in full view. If you think your partner may feel uncomfortable, reassure her that you love her body, or don't encourage her to put herself in a vulnerable position. She may be more comfortable in this position keeping a pretty bra or teddy on.

TIPS

➤ To increase the odds of coming during intercourse or coming with her, stimulate her clitoris to the point where she is about to orgasm, then get into the woman-superior position. If you thrust, there is a good chance she'll be able to reach orgasm with you inside of her (Position C, facing toward you).

➤ She can stimulate the G-spot area of her front vaginal wall, and if you love her butt, you can play with it.

➤ Position B is only good if a man's erection will flex this way. It's often not very good for younger, tight-to-the-tummy guys. But it is great for a couple who enjoy anal play. If she leans forward and has her chest on his legs, he can stroke her anus and perineal area and she can be in her own world.

SIDE BY SIDE

For this position, the man and woman are on their sides with their legs entwined like scissors. You can be facing each other or you can be behind her. The beauty of side by side is that most men can thrust for a long time in this position without climaxing. It provides couples the opportunity to make their intimate encounter last. And because penetration is not as deep in this position, women who have lovers with exceptionally large penises say that intercourse is more comfortable. Much like in the man-superior position, kissing and hugging are almost inevitable here.

Position A shows the true scissors of the legs; now all you have to do is lift your upper leg and have her drop onto the bed. Now you have a totally new position, in which you will be able to manually play with her clitoral area or breasts. In this "X" position, you can keep your hands joined together and use them to create your thrusting pelvic motions.

In Position B, she has wrapped her legs firmly around him and can keep him in as closely as she likes during his movements.

Position C is good for spooning, which allows a man easy access to her entire body. Perhaps the best thing about making love side by side, however, is that it is the one position that lends itself to falling asleep comfortably in each other's arms afterward.

Side by Side

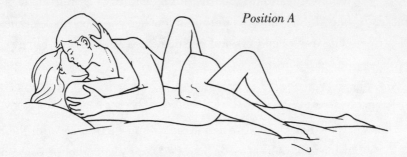

Position A

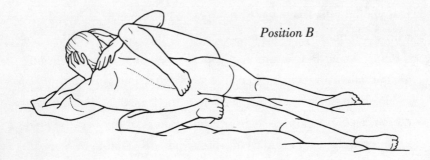

Position B

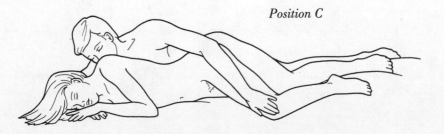

Position C

There is a variation on Position C, again for the more athletic. This is how it's done:

Step 1: The man is inside the woman, penetrating from behind. She places her upper leg close to her chest or between her breasts.

Step 2: While maintaining penetration, the man shifts his position from behind her so that he's more on top of the woman's hip. Now all of his weight will be balanced between her hips and his knees. Because his hands are not supporting him, they are now free to create more sensation and stimulation from behind.

Step 3: Assuming she is on her left side, he can insert the pinkie finger of his left hand into her anus (just a little, and it is best to start conservatively with this motion). While he gently inserts his right thumb into her vagina to increase the width sensation for her, he can use his right hand's index finger to stimulate the clitoral region.

TIPS

➤ When you are positioned behind her, you can also stimulate her clitoris.

➤ Rear entry in side-to-side position can be good for pregnant women, as she will be able to support her abdomen and he can play with her full breasts, assuming she likes this.

MALE FROM BEHIND
(AKA DOGGY STYLE)

Many women have said that the male-from-behind or doggy-style position makes for some of their most erotic sex. Men as well find this position highly charged. Women have said their reasons range from the intense depth of penetration to the feeling of being taken. Some women also enjoy the speed that a man can create by holding onto

Man from Behind

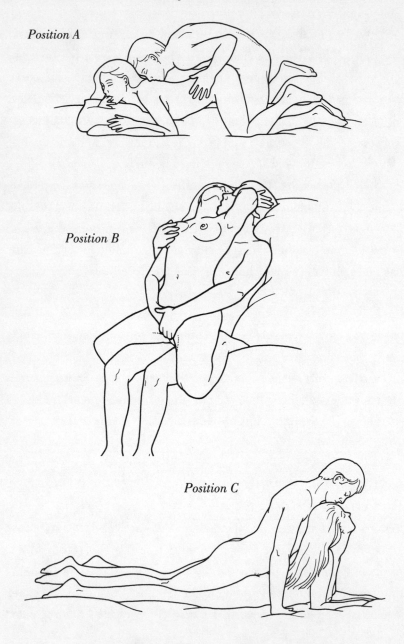

Position A

Position B

Position C

her hips and thrusting, creating momentum. Then again, a man can control the speed of his thrusting if a woman enjoys variation or slow thrusting.

Women who have given birth have an increased sensitivity to G-spot stimulation in this position. Since their vaginas are more elastic, the G-spot is more reachable by the penis.

This position can be done with the woman lying flat on her stomach, which allows for a tight entry with a feeling of being taken (C). Other options are: the woman on all fours (A), the woman standing up bent over at the waist, or the woman lying on her side with her back to her lover. The man enters her vagina from the back of her rather than from in front of her. That's why it is often referred to as rear-entry sex. Men say this is the position in which they experience the most heat, created by the touching of her crotch and butt against his thighs. (FYI: Backdoor sex is anal sex.)

In Position A, men can kiss down her back. And again, pillows can come in very handy for under the chest. Position B gives the man full access to her body and she can feel the heat of him and relax into the sensations. She can also extend her legs down to create more thrusting capability.

SECRET FROM LOU'S ARCHIVES

Position B is a fun position for the beach. Slip the thong to the side, and away you go.

TIPS
➤ The only drawback to rear-entry sex is that because it is so highly erotic, men often reach their climax more quickly than they do in other positions.

- This position can be painful if a woman has a tilted uterus or a very large partner, because he will likely hit the neck of her cervix.
- You can be stimulating her with your hands as you penetrate her.

SECRET FROM LOU'S ARCHIVES

As a male dentist told me, "This position smells more of sex; and I love the animalness of it."

STANDING UP

For the sake of balance, this position is best done with the woman standing against a wall and the man standing in front of her unless he is particularly strong. The shower and pool are often not as nifty settings as one would like—for one main reason: The natural lubrication is washed away and therefore thrusting is made tougher, not easier, by the water. Standing positions work better when you have the lady in a recumbent (lying down) position. You can use the strongest muscles in your body, your glutes and thighs, to their greatest advantage. Though another position is probably best for a long romantic sexual encounter, this one is excellent for hot and urgent sex or athletic sex. In its simplest form, try both of you standing. This can be done without the complete removal of clothes (a plus when you're both in a hurry) and requires very little space to do it in.

Position A shows a variation on the woman-on-the-table theme. Once you have entered her, gentlemen, hold on to her hips and place the back of her heels on your shoulders, so her hips and open labia are flush against you. Men have stated that they get a great view and more scent, rather like the rear entry in reverse. Her back should be

Standing Up

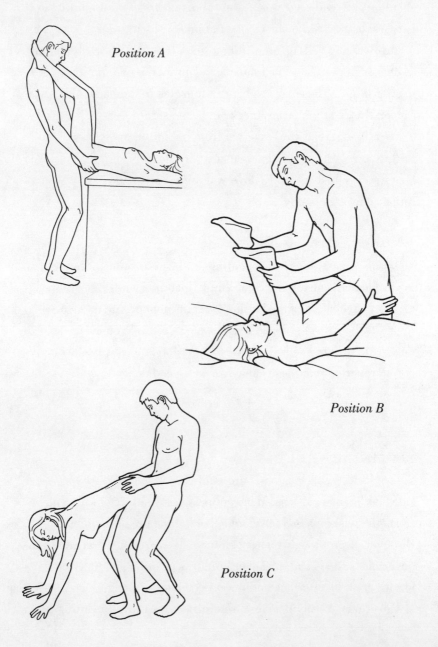

Position A

Position B

Position C

in a straight line. This is easiest if she locks her heels over your shoulders. Why does it work? Your penis is stroking very firmly over her G-spot area while she can be manually playing with her clitoris.

In Position B, the man is able to see all of her sex and penetrate as deeply as possible. The woman can control his penetration by flexing her thighs. These are the biggest muscles in the body. The variation on this is to place her knees out to the side.

I call Position C the "take her from behind in the garden." Great for quickies! One man commented, "She has these great mirrored doors in her hallway and I love watching her breasts sway while I thrust. That's the ticket!"

TIPS
➤ If you are doing this standing up, be sure your knees are locked and you are comfortably leaning against a solid wall. I have heard of men falling over at inopportune moments.
➤ If the lady is going to wrap her legs around you, hang on. Make sure she has removed her stilettos. It has been reported that these can cause serious damage to calf muscles.

SITTING/KNEELING

Sitting or kneeling positions are simply a variation of the side-by-side and facing positions. Many couples enjoy sitting or kneeling because the positions feel novel and give them a break in their routine. However, even though some positions have a reduced range of motion, unless she is standing over him, this position generally does allow for great face-to-face and/or body contact.

Positions A and B give a whole new meaning to dining room

Sitting and Kneeling

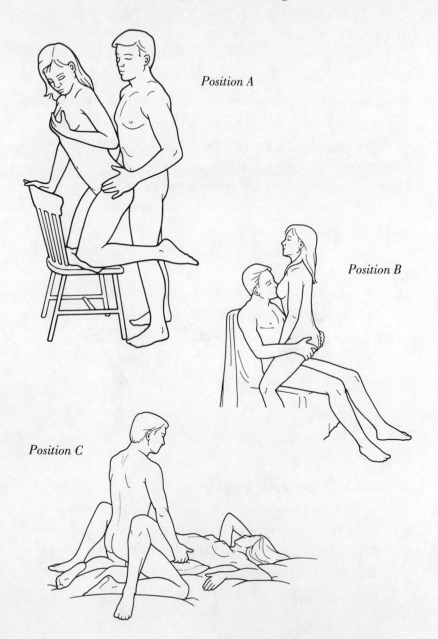

Position A

Position B

Position C

chairs. In A the lady needs to hold on to the chair so she's balanced—or you could thrust her right off the chair. This allows her the greatest range of hip motion while he remains still.

In Position C, his thighs support the backs of her legs and she has a pillow under her hips to keep her at the right level for entry. Meanwhile, you hold her hips to keep her in as close as possible. Your thrusting will likely cause her breasts to jiggle, an often enjoyable sight. A variation is to place the back of her knees in the crook of your elbow, like a barbell curl position. By doing "curls" with your entire arm, not only will she see your hard work from the gym, you'll experience internal glans stimulation and she'll have internal G-spot zone stimulation.

TIPS

➤ Sitting, she can be straddling you, facing away while seated on your lap, or facing sideways in your lap.

➤ An easy position to move to from the woman-superior position; the woman pulls her legs forward and the man can sit up.

➤ Sitting on a chair is good for couples who want a quickie or if the woman is pregnant.

GENERAL TIPS FOR INTERCOURSE

➤ If you experience a burning sensation during intercourse, check to see if you need more lubricant or if you mistakenly used a lubricant with nonoxynol-9. If neither of these is a possible explanation, you may want to visit your doctor and check for an infection or STD. She may be having an allergic reaction to your semen.

- If your partner complains of pain during intercourse, your penis may be hitting the neck of her cervix or uterus; try changing your position. You may also be irritating episiotomy scars or, again, an STD-induced soreness.
- Regardless of how much you exercise and how many different techniques and positions you put into your sexual repertoire, just remember that the single most important factor in determining your level of sexual fulfillment during intercourse will be the release of your inhibitions and wanting to be with her.

The Best Pregnancy Positions

Mother Nature never intended for us to stop having sex when women are pregnant. Some women report their best sex ever is during their pregnancies; some women can't take it at all. The lesson: Ask her how she feels. One woman said, "I'd love to go back to pregnant sex. I could come so easily. Now, ten months after the fact, it's much

---

SECRET FROM LOU'S ARCHIVES

As a physician said, there should be three sexes: women, pregnant women, and men. Pregnant women are as different from nonpregnant women as they are from men.

---

harder." On the other hand, there are those women who, because of terrible morning sickness or general physical discomfort, may not want you penetrating her. Again, in this case, it's very much up to her. In general, male and female superior are fine in the early months of a pregnancy, but as the woman's stomach enlarges, these positions become more and more difficult. In later stages of pregnancy, side by side (Positions A and C) and sitting and kneeling (Positions A and B) all work well. In this case, you are not on top, but still close-in. The classic spooning position side by side (C) works well because her tummy is supported and deep penetration is not possible. For very late-stage pregnancy, some prefer the sitting positions—either facing sideways or toward one another, depending on the size of the woman's tummy.

Anal Penetration

Some women love it, some women hate it. Like swallowing your semen, there tends to be no in-between when it comes to how women feel and experience anal sex. Women are either in one camp or the other. Most women have tried anal sex at least once (usually because their partner has suggested it). Women who love being penetrated in this way claim that the sensation is intense.

Part of the reluctance of men and women to the very idea of anal sex is its negative associations. According to Tristan Taormino in her book *The Ultimate Guide to Anal Sex for Women*, there are ten pervasive yet inaccurate myths about anal sex:

1. It's unnatural and amoral.
2. Only sluts, perverts, and weirdos have anal sex.
3. The anus and rectum were not meant to be eroticized.
4. Anal sex is dirty and messy.
5. Only gay men have anal sex.
6. Straight men who like anal sex must be homosexual.

7. Anal sex is painful.
8. Women don't enjoy receiving anal sex; they do it just to please their partners.
9. Anal sex is the easiest way to get AIDS.
10. Anal sex is naughty.

These attitudes toward anal sex are tied to outdated and moralistic beliefs that sex is meant only for procreation, which also implies that sex shouldn't be enjoyed. As far as I am concerned, nothing could be further from the truth. Sex is not only meant to give two people a way to express their love and commitment through deep pleasure; it's also a manner of human expression that should never be judged outright. If it doesn't hurt, then it's perfectly natural and essentially good.

Some women like being anally penetrated while they are also being stimulated clitorally. For other women, the intensity of anal penetration is too overwhelming, making it impossible for them to climax. One reason it is difficult to enjoy anal play is the fact that there are actually two sphincters that need to be relaxed. As I pointed out earlier, one sphincter is under voluntary control and the other is under involuntary control, which, no matter how much you try, is impossible to consciously relax. A good way to try to relax the anus is to insert one finger for one minute, two fingers for two minutes. I also suggest lubricating generously, as this is not a self-lubricating area. Consider asking your partner to bear down, which will relax the sphincters and ease entry.

TIPS
➤ The best position for rear entry is shoulders down, pillow underneath. You can massage her anus with your thumb.
➤ Another good position is her on her back with her legs rolled

forward, with a pillow under her hips. She can hook her forearms under her thighs to increase the curve and give you more access to her anus.

➤ Do not return to vaginal intercourse until you have washed your penis or changed your condom; otherwise you risk giving each other an infection.

➤ Removing the finger/toy/penis should be done *very* slowly!

A Final Note

In my years of working with and listening to men and women about their sexuality, I have learned that having great sex is tied to being an artful, fearless, and adventurous lover. Therefore, while the techniques, positions, and hints I have provided you with in this book will make you technically proficient, being an expert lover is much more about your attitude. It's about feeling confident and trusting yourself. It's about wanting to please your lover. It's about really caring.

I have also learned in my years of working with men and women that the deepest and most satisfying sex usually comes when two people are open, honest, and respectful in their communication. Once these principles are in place, there are no bounds to the passion, spontaneity, and wonderful, soul-merging sex you and your partner can experience. And I offer you this book in hopes that it brings you to that joyful, fun place with your lover. Enjoy!

Bibliography

═══════ • ═══════

Anand, Margo. *The Art of Sexual Ecstasy: The Path of Sacred Sexuality for Western Lovers.* 450 pp. Jeremy Tarcher, Los Angeles. 1989.

―――――. *The Art of Sexual Magic: Cultivating Sexual Energy to Transform Your Life.* 383 pp. Tarcher/Putnam, New York. 1995.

Bakos, Susan Crain. *What Men Really Want: Straight Talk from Men About Sex.* 225 pp. St. Martin's, New York. 1990.

Barbach, Lonnie. *For Each Other: Sharing Sexual Intimacy.* 305 pp. Anchor, New York. 1982.

Barrows, Sydney Biddle. *Mayflower Manners: Etiquette for Consenting Adults.* 221 pp. Doubleday, New York. 1990.

Bechtel, Stefan. *The Practical Encyclopedia of Sex and Health.* 366 pp. Rodale, Emmaus, PA. 1993.

―――――. *Sex: A Man's Guide.* 500 pp. Rodale, Emmaus, PA. 1996.

Birch, Robert. *Oral Caress: The Loving Guide to Exciting a Woman: A Comprehensive Illustrated Manual on the Joyful Art of Cunnilingus.* 138 pp. PEC Publications, Columbus, OH. 1996.

Bishop, Clifford. *Sex and Spirit.* 184 pp. Little, Brown, New York. 1996.

Blank, Joani. *Good Vibrations: The Complete Guide to Vibrators.* 70 pp. Down There Press, San Francisco. 1989.

Brothers, Joyce. *What Every Woman Should Know About Men.* 218 pp. Simon & Schuster, New York. 1981.

Caine, K. Winston. *The Male Body: An Owner's Manual.* 405 pp. Rodale, Emmaus, PA. 1996.

Chesser, Eustace. *Strange Loves: The Human Aspects of Sexual Deviation.* 255 pp. William Morrow, New York. 1971.

Chichester, B., ed. *Sex Secrets: Ways to Satisfy Your Partner Every Time*. 168 pp. Rodale, Emmaus, PA. 1996.

Cohen, Angela, and Fox, Sarah Gardner. *The Wise Woman's Guide to Erotic Videos: 300 Sexy Videos for Every Woman—and Her Lover*. 296 pp. Broadway, New York. 1997.

Comfort, Alex. *The Joy of Sex: A Gourmet Guide to Love Making*. 253 pp. Fireside/Simon & Schuster, New York. 1972.

———. *The New Joy of Sex: A Gourmet Guide to Lovemaking for the Nineties*. 256 pp. Crown, New York. 1991.

Danielou, Alain. *The Complete Kama Sutra*. 560 pp. Park Street Press, VT. 1994.

Deida, David. *The Way of the Superior Lover: A Spiritual Guide to the Sexual Skills*. 131 pp. Plexus, TX. 1997.

Dick & Jane. *Erotic New York: A Guide to the Red Hot Apple*. 144 pp. City & Company, New York. 1997.

Dodson, Betty. *Sex for One: The Joy of Self-Loving*. 191 pp. Crown, New York. 1996.

Douglas, Nik, and Slinger, Penny. *Sexual Secrets: The Alchemy of Ecstasy*. 10th Anniversary Issue. 383 pp. Destiny Books, VT. 1989.

Eichel, Edward, and Nobile, Philip. *The Perfect Fit: How to Achieve Mutual Fulfillment and Monogamous Passion Through the New Intercourse*. 238 pp. Signet, New York. 1993.

Estes, Clarissa Pinkola. *Women Who Run with the Wolves: Myths and Stories of the Wild Woman Archetype*. 537 pp. Ballantine, New York. 1992.

Fisher, Helen. *Anatomy of Love: The Natural History of Monogamy, Adultery and Divorce*. 431 pp. W. W. Norton, New York. 1992.

———. *The First Sex: The Natural Talents of Women and How They Are Changing the World*. 378 pp. Random House, New York. 1999.

George, Stephen C. *A Lifetime of Sex: The Ultimate Manual on Sex, Women and Relationships for Every Stage of a Man's Life*. 578 pp. Rodale, Emmaus, PA. 1998.

Gerstman, Bradley, Pizzo, Christopher, and Seldes, Bradley. *What Men Really Want: Three Professional Men Reveal to Women What It Takes to Make a Man Yours*. 204 pp. Cliff Street Books/HarperCollins, New York. 1998.

Gordon, Sol. *The New You*. 242 pp. An Ed-U Press, Fayetteville, NY. 1980.

Gray, John. *Mars and Venus in the Bedroom: A Guide to Lasting Romance and Passion*. 206 pp. HarperCollins, New York. 1995.

———. *Men, Women and Relationships: Making Peace with the Opposite Sex.* 226 pp. Beyond Words Publishing, Hillsboro, OR. 1993.

Griffin, Gary. *The Condom Encyclopedia.* 128 pp. Added Dimensions, Los Angeles. 1993.

Harris, Marvin. *Our Kind: Who We Are, Where We Came From and Where We Are Going.* 548 pp. Harper & Row, New York. 1989.

Hatcher, Robert A. *Contraceptive Technology.* 16th ed. 730 pp. Irvington Publishers, New York. 1994.

Heimel, Cynthia. *Sex Tips for Girls.* 205 pp. Simon & Schuster, New York. 1983.

Hite, Shere. *The Hite Report: A Nationwide Study on Female Sexuality.* 638 pp. Dell, New York. 1976.

———. *The Hite Report: On Male Sexuality.* 1053 pp. Ballantine, New York. 1981.

Hollander, Xaviera. *The Happy Hooker.* 311 pp. Dell, New York. 1972.

Hutton, Julia. *Good Sex: Real Stories from Real People.* 227 pp. Cleis Press, San Francisco. 1995.

J. *The Sensuous Woman.* 192 pp. Dell, New York. 1969.

Janus, Samuel, and Janus, Cynthia. *The Janus Report on Sexual Behavior: The First Broad-Scale Scientific National Survey Since Kinsey.* 430 pp. John Wiley, New York. 1993.

Joannides, Paul. *The Guide to Getting It On: A New and Mostly Wonderful Book About Sex.* 368 pp. Goofy Foot Press, Los Angeles. 1996.

Kahn, Alice, Whipple, Beverly, and Perry, John. *The G Spot: and Other Recent Discoveries About Human Sexuality.* 236 pp. Dell, New York. 1982.

Kahn, Sandra. *The Kahn Report on Sexual Preferences.* 278 pp. Avon, New York. 1981.

Kaplan, Helen Singer. *The New Sex Therapy: The Active Treatment of Sexual Disorders.* 544 pp. Brunner/Mazel, New York. 1974.

Keesling, Barbara. *How to Make Love All Night (and Drive a Woman Wild). Male Multiple Orgasm and Other Secrets for Prolonging Lovemaking.* 178 pp. Harper Perennial, New York. 1994.

Kline-Graber, Georgia, and Graber, Benjamin. *A Guide to Sexual Satisfaction: Woman's Orgasm.* 240 pp. Popular Library, New York. 1976.

Kronhausen, Phyllis, and Kronehausen, Eberhard. *The Complete Book of Erotic Art*, vols. 1 and 2. 582 pp. Bell Publishing, New York. 1978.

Legman, G. *The Intimate Kiss: The Modern Classic of Oral Erotic Technique.* 286 pp. Warner, New York. 1973.

Lewinsohn, Richard. *A History of Sexual Customs.* 424 pp. Harper & Brothers, New York. 1958.

Locker, Sari. *Mindblowing Sex in the Real World: Hot Tips for Doing It in the Age of Anxiety.* 258 pp. HarperPerennial, New York. 1995.

Love, Brenda. *Encyclopedia of Unusual Sex Practices.* 336 pp. Barricade Books, New York. 1992.

M. *The Sensuous Man.* 216 pp. Dell, New York, 1971.

Mann, A. T., and Lyle, Jane. *Sacred Sexuality.* 192 pp. Element Books, England. 1995.

Massey, Doreen. *Lovers' Guide Encyclopedia: The Definitive Guide to Sex and You.* 256 pp. Thunder's Mouth Press, New York. 1996.

Masters, William; Johnson, Virginia; and Kolodny, Robert C. *Heterosexuality.* 595 pp. HarperCollins, New York. 1994.

McCary, James Leslie. *Sexual Myths & Fallacies.* 206 pp. Schocken, New York. 1973.

Morris, Hugh. *The Art of Kissing.* 47 pp. 1936.

Muir, Charles, and Muir, Caroline. *Tantra: The Art of Conscious Loving.* 134 pp. Mercury House, San Francisco. 1989.

Neret, Gilles. *Erotica Universalis.* 756 pp. Benedikt Taschen Verlag, Germany. 1994.

Panati, Charles. *Sexy Origins and Intimate Things: The Rites and Rituals of Straights, Gays, Bi's, Drags, Trans, Virgins and Others.* 526 pp. Penguin Books, New York. 1998.

Parsons, Alexandra. *Facts & Phalluses: A Collection of Bizarre and Intriguing Truths, Legends and Measurements.* 84 pp. St. Martin's, New York. 1990.

Patterson, Ella. *Will the Real Women . . . Please Stand Up!* 220 pp. Knowledge Concepts, TX. 1993.

Penney, Alexandra. *The Sexiest Sex of All.* 145 pp. Dell, New York. 1993.

Purvis, Kenneth. *The Male Sexual Machine: An Owner's Manual.* 210 pp. St. Martin's, New York. 1992.

Ramsdale, David, and Dorfman, Ellen. *Sexual Energy Ecstasy.* 380 pp. Peak Skill Publishing, Playa del Rey, CA. 1991.

Reinsch, Judith. *The Kinsey Institute New Report on Sex: What You Must Know to Be Sexually Literate.* 540 pp. St. Martin's, New York. 1990.

Sacks, Stephen. *The Truth About Herpes,* 4th ed. 316 pp. Gordon Soules Publishers Ltd., Vancouver. 1997.

SARK. *Succulent Wild Women: Dancing with Your Wonder-full Self!* 180 pp. Fireside/Simon & Schuster, New York. 1997.

Schnarch, David. *Passionate Couples: Love, Sex and Intimacy in Emotionally Committed Relationships.* 432 pp. W. W. Norton, New York. 1997.

Scoble, Gretchen, and Field, Ann. *The Meaning of Flowers: Myth, Language and Lore.* 108 pp. Chronicle Books, San Francisco. 1998.

Smith, David, and Gordon, Mike. *Strange but True Facts about Sex: The Illustrated Book of Sexual Trivia.* 64 pp. Meadowbook Press, MN. 1989.

Stoppard, Miriam. *The Magic of Sex: The Book That Really Tells Men About Women and Women About Men.* 256 pp. Dorling Kindersley, New York. 1991.

Stubbs, Kenneth Ray, and Saulnier, Louise-Andrée. *Erotic Massage: The Touch of Love.* 112 pp. Secret Garden, Larkspur CA. 1993.

Tannahill, Reay. *Sex in History.* 480 pp. Scarborough House, Briarcliff Manor, NY. 1980.

Tannen, Deborah. *You Just Don't Understand: Women and Men in Conversation.* 330 pp. William Morrow, New York, 1990.

Taormino, Tristan. *The Ultimate Guide to Anal Sex for Women.* 151 pp. Cleis Press, San Francisco. 1998.

Taylor, Timothy. *The Prehistory of Sex: Four Million Years of Human Sexual Culture.* 356 pp. Bantam, New York. 1996.

Trager, James. *The Women's Chronology: A Year-by-Year Record, from Prehistory to the Present.* 787 pp. Henry Holt, New York. 1994.

Tuleja, Tad. *Curious Customs: The Stories Behind 296 Popular American Rituals.* 210 pp. Harmony Books/Crown, New York. 1987.

Waggoner, Glen, and Moloney, Kathleen. *Esquire Etiquette: The Modern Man's Guide to Good Form.* 180 pp. Collier Books, New York. 1987.

Walker, Morton. *Foods for Fabulous Sex: Natural Sexual Nutrients to Trigger Passion, Heighten Response, Improve Performance and Overcome Dysfunction.* 160 pp. Magni Group, TX. 1992.

Watson, Cynthia Mervis. *Love Potions: A Guide to Aphrodisiacs and Sexual Pleasures.* 272 pp. Tarcher/Putnam, New York. 1993.

Welch, Leslee. *Sex Facts: A Handbook for the Carnally Curious.* 100 pp. Carol, New York. 1992.

Wildwood, Chrissie. *Erotic Aromatherapy: Essential Oils for Lovers.* 160 pp. Sterling, New York. 1994.

Worwood, Valerie Ann. *Scents and Scentuality: Aromatherapy and Essential Oils for Romance, Love and Sex.* 234 pp. New World Library, Novato, CA. 1999.

Zilbergeld, Bernie. *Male Sexuality.* 411 pp. Bantam, New York. 1978.

———. *New Male Sexuality: The Truth About Men, Sex and Pleasure.* 580 pp. Bantam, New York. 1992.

Zimet, Susan, and Goodman, Victor. *The Great Cover-up: A Condom Compendium.* 121 pp. Civan, New York. 1988.